A Self-Help Manual
On
Cosmeticus Interruptus
How to perform it &
why you need to

CONFESSIONS
Of A
COSMETIC
DENTIST

ALAN S JAY D.D.S
World's Best Cosmetic Dentist

Pumping Irony Press

The opinions expressed in this manuscript are solely the opinions of the author and do not represent the opinions or thoughts of the publisher. The author has represented and warranted full ownership and/or legal right to publish all the materials in this book.

Confessions Of A Cosmetic Dentist
A Self-Help Manual On Cosmeticus Interruptus
How to perform it & why you need to
All Rights Reserved.
Copyright © 2014 Alan S Jay D.D.S., W.B.C.D.
v3.0

Cover Photo © 2014 JupiterImages Corporation. All rights reserved - used with permission.

This book may not be reproduced, transmitted, or stored in whole or in part by any means, including graphic, electronic, or mechanical without the express written consent of the publisher except in the case of brief quotations embodied in critical articles and reviews.

Pumping Irony Press

ISBN: 978-0-578-13720-9

Library of Congress Control Number: 2014902590

PRINTED IN THE UNITED STATES OF AMERICA

To Rose and Sidney

"If they ask me I could write a book"
Lyrics from "I Could Write a Book"...Rogers & Hart

They didn't, I did anyway...Alan S Jay WBCD

truth is the safest lie
Maxwell Carver 1988 Contributing Editor DISCOVER

ACKNOWLEDGEMENTS

It was my mother who told me 'never speak unless spoken to', advice that with few exceptions I've virtually ignored.

What needs to be acknowledged, that shouldn't be ignored, is that whether you take mine about cosmetic recommendations 'pushed' on you by anyone other than the World's Best Cosmetic Dentist (that would be me), *'the worst that could happen' (that would be to you) will be to write a check for more than you ever imagined in exchange for elective treatment that was disguised as a necessity. The consolation for not being disappointed with the 'ends' doesn't justify any of your doctor's 'means' for getting you there.

I'll give you this; while the majority of my cosmetically persuaded peers are capable of significantly improving your 'face value', there are a few things you should keep in mind:

1. Just because they can doesn't mean you ought to let them.
2. If you already have, they just might have me to thank.
3. If after you read the book and decide not to let them?
4. You can thank me, because they certainly won't.
5. You're welcome.

*Johnny Maestro and the Crests from 'The Worst That Could Happen' released 1968

PROLOGUE

Life is what happens while you're planning for the future.

John Lennon was right; there are no warning signs to prepare you for the unexpected. If you're luckier than he was, there IS a life after an untimely interruption, which is how I got a new one when "COSMETICUS INTERRUPTUS" changed mine.

Practicing, lecturing, and once again divorcing, the furthest thing from my mind on that sunny day in May was thinking about what my "last one" in the office would feel like.

Speaking of "lasts," the only other day that came to mind was the one from a lifetime ago when my accountant was setting up an IRA with a formula that would give me enough money to comfortably retire on when it was time.; Retirement, the time I was supposed to be looking forward to, when I'd be free to pursue those "other interests," whatever they were.

I decided then and there that when my time was up, it would be scripted with a Hollywood ending. It would be a walk-off homerun; a final rounding of the bases in celebration of a professional career which the record would show was deserving of Hall of Fame consideration.

I could close my eyes and just imagine it; my entire dental team awaiting me as I rounded third and headed for home, unable to contain their enthusiasm with their congratulations as we all shared the fitting storybook ending to a distinguished career.

As it would turn out, unbeknownst to me, my last "at bat" had already been entered in the record books.

It was the end of that December day as I finished up with the final patient, lingering longer than usual to chat with my chair-side dental assistant before retreating to the sanctuary of my private office and sinking into the leather chair behind my desk.

I went over it once again, The Plan I'd put together with my staff to keep everything going until my rescheduled return exactly six weeks later.

"Don't worry, just leave it to us, the practice will be fine, we'll be fine, and so will you."

The neurosurgeon had predicted that while I should be back to my old self by then, there would be some things I might not be able to do as well as before.

ME: "As well as before?" I wasn't worried. I planned on doing them better.

I left the office for the nearby airport and a flight to NYC to undergo what would be a fifteen-hour surgery to remove a brain tumor. One of those unexpected outcomes diagnosed from a "precautionary MRI" that my ENT physician and good friend expected would rule out anything to worry about after I complained about a slight hearing loss in my right ear except where to go for the smallest hearing aid in existence.

That tomorrow would come is predictable; it was the tomorrow after brain surgery that I couldn't count on.

I recall waking up post-surgery in the ICU, where I would stay for another week.

As predicted, I could do most things better than before save one glaring exception.

It's a recurring bad dream, one in which I make that sensational career culminating walk-off homerun, only to discover that unlike the promise of John Fogerty's "Centerfield" there's only the echo of an empty ballpark "as I'm rounding third headed for home."

It's my paraphrased Browning quote that best describes it:

"Look to this day, for it is life; in its brief course lies the verities and realities of your existence, for yesterday is but a dream, and tomorrow... only a vision," and the day to start writing a book.

So I did.

Read The Book!
If for no other reason than they don't want you to

The last straw was being told what an "inexcusable error in judgment" it would be to make available more information than what patients need to know about how cosmetic dentistry is sold because it would only "confuse" them.

I doubt you'll be confused by what you're about to read; more likely you'll be better informed.

It's not complicated.
Everyone knows more is better.

If anything is "inexcusable," it would be not publishing the book sooner. As for making excuses, start by asking those who promised I'd live to regret it if I ever did what theirs are for not wanting you to read it.

Once you do, the only thing you'll regret is accepting a cosmetic treatment recommendation without first applying reasonable doubt.

While second thoughts are invariably wiser, exercising them to question your dentist's wisdom will invariably make you less popular.

I wasn't expecting to win a popularity contest when I wrote it, nor should you once you apply it.

Carl Icahn said it best:

If you need a friend, get a dog.

CONTENTS

Acknowledgements i
Prologue iii
Read The Book! vii

I. INTRODUCTION
WHAT TO EXPECT FROM THE WORLD'S BEST

Chapter One: What You Know For Sure That Just Isn't So 1
Chapter Two: Sex, Lies, & Tales from the Oral Cavity 4
Chapter Three: Better Safe than Sorry 12
Chapter Four: Why NO Means Not Yet 22
Chapter Five: Familiarity That Borders On Contempt 24
Chapter Six: Respect, I Get No Respect At All 28
Chapter Seven: Veni, Vidi, Video 36
Chapter Eight: Is It Safe? 43
Chapter Nine: Finders Keepers, Referrers Weepers 53
Chapter Ten: When the Cover-Up IS Office Policy 60
Chapter Eleven: Making a List, Checking It Twice… 69
Chapter Twelve: Insider Trading Without the Risk 78
Chapter Thirteen: Foreplay That Puts a Smile on Your Face 80
Chapter Fourteen: Leave No Smile Behind 85
Chapter Fifteen: Encore, Anyone? 87
Chapter Sixteen: It's Not Complicated 88
Chapter Seventeen: FOR DENTISTS ONLY 93
Epilogue: The Final Confession 104
Author's Note 107
Definitions You Won't Find Anywhere Else But Here 109

I. INTRODUCTION

What To Expect From The World's Best

There was never a time when I didn't aspire to be the best that I could be, long before the Armed Forces issued the challenge. No one asked, no one told, and in spite of all those telling me to stop, no one could, until I stopped myself.

When the aspiration for being "discovered" didn't happen in my first six months as the lead singer in a rock & roll band, it was time to leave the stage and face the music. I pulled out of the tour, pulled out the plug to my Fender, and stuck a pin in my music balloon to let the air out of my dream.

I (STILL) WANTED TO BE A ROCK STAR
(What comebacks are all about?)
BUT MY FATHER CONVINCED ME
THAT WOMEN WORSHIP DOCTORS

I took his advice, went back to school, and after graduating at the top of my class decided that the best thing for me to be would be a dentist.

I've met several rock & roll artists who wished they'd gone to dental school; I'm the only one I know who actually did and one who saw his aspirations of becoming the World's Best Cosmetic Dentist come true.

After realizing my dreams and living them for twenty-five years, the call of the unknown beckoned. No matter that I loved what I did every day I did it; I couldn't resist the temptation of taking the road less traveled.

Whoever came up with the idea that "nothing is as permanent as change itself" had something. As I agonized over how best to deliver my next "act," an idea took root, no pun intended, for leveling the playing field.

It starts by giving you an insider's glimpse of how the cosmetically persuaded dentist sells his patients on the idea that "life will look better when they do' for getting his treatment recommendation accepted.

The convincing aside, I want you to know that the majority of the persuadees I've come in contact with over my years in practice have convinced themselves that the benefits of Appearance Dentistry for their patients justifies whatever it takes to push it.

In the hope of avoiding persecution as well as potential prosecution for disclosing the privileged insider information you need to know for pushing back, I've published this book under an assumed name. I've written it in semi-nonfiction, my homegrown tenderizer for softening the truth to make it easier for you to digest.

I've chosen to educate you with an eclectic collection of the good, the bad, and the dysfunctional practices I used for promoting Cosmetic Dentistry to my patients that dentists enrolling in my seminars imitated and took back to their offices to use on theirs. Never underestimate the value of applying a sense of humor for helping you understand and see things that defy logic; and humor is what you'll need after you use my checklist for grading your dentist's standard of care.

Thomas Alva Edison is credited with saying: "The value of an idea lies in the using of it."

It's not complicated, fail to use these ideas and you've got a lot more to lose than you think.

Alan S Jay DDS WBCD

Cosmeticus Interruptus:

n. The affirmative action taken for denying any dentist the satisfaction of 'having you (accept his cosmetic treatment presentation) at hello'.

Accomplished by physically pulling (one's self) out of a case presentation for a strategic time-out to gain some objectivity from your 'second thoughts that will be invariably wiser' in overcoming the uncontrollable urge to give in to his heretofore seductive recommendations when you return.

alt. an elective interruption in a dentist's practice of Cosmetic Dentistry; recusing himself from recommending and performing smile makeovers to pursue other interests.

Second thoughts are invariably wiser.
Euripides 480-405 B.C.
Greek playwright

CHAPTER ONE

What You Know For Sure That Just Isn't So

1. Why you're being pushed into Cosmetic Dentistry

Cosmetic Dentistry got its roots, so to speak, when the added value of "pushing" it became the logical solution to reverse what had become a nationwide trend of decreasing profitability, which for the most part was due to the increasing numbers of patients getting dental insurance. Making matters worse, the holes in the appointment books that dentists were dealing with on a daily basis were becoming sleepless nights of worrying about how to fill them.

What many of them did was make the decision to accept dental insurance, and those who did were signing up for more.

Dentists became "providers," the insurance company designation for a doctor who is under contract to provide treatment to their qualified policy holders. Provided, that is, he accept being paid less than his standard fee in order to provide them with as much profit as possible.

As more patients qualified for dental insurance with their employment benefit package, increasing numbers of dentists were invited to become "preferred providers," soon discovering how much faster they had to work in order to make up for providing more services for more patients under a revised preferred fee schedule that paid them less. It's not complicated—reading the fine print would have been better.

It was out of necessity—being the mother of invention—that the profession needed to invent (if you will) a service that dental insurance couldn't determine reimbursement for.

Almost overnight the push to perform COSMETIC DENTISTRY exploded.

Suddenly advertisements and commercials extolling the virtues of recapturing a more youthful appearance by improving your smile began to appear.

Many dental associations were pressured by their members to subsidize advertising campaigns extolling the benefits not just of healthy teeth and gums but the importance of an attractive smile for improving the "quality of life."

It was now "in" to ask your dentist, if he wasn't already asking you, what to do to get *it*. And 'it' was plastic surgery without the scalpel.

If you didn't say uncle to the argument that a Hollywood smile would give you a critical leg up on your quest for personal and professional success, your dentist was learning better ways of twisting your arm to convince you.

Cosmetic Dentistry was Push Merchandise without the inventory. Unlike boxes carefully marked with a PM stamp at the shoe boutique that a salesman could earn a significant extra commission for pushing a customer out the door with, every elective cosmetic procedure was a self-contained PM box in itself.

The demand for Appearance Dentistry (term courtesy of the WBCD) increased proportionately with the emphasis of dentists pushing it, which is precisely what they were doing because it was more profitable, not to mention a vast improvement over pushing out the pages of insurance claim forms for services they were providing at a discount.

In hopes of attracting a more cosmetically inclined and less insurance dependent clientele, general dentists underwent a metamorphosis and emerged as Doctors of Cosmetic Dentistry, or at least that's what the explosion of new office signs replacing General Dentistry pronounced.

Numbers of dentists joined newly formed cosmetic organizations for no other purpose than to list them on their resumes and prominently display the membership plaques on their office walls.

To prosper required a new game plan, and pushing cosmetics was the new kid on the block.

I promise you that there isn't a single dentist who has ever attended one of my courses who didn't learn that success in selling elective cosmetic treatment requires giving patients a push in the intended direction.

Jack Nicholson was right as rain and right on the money when he said: "The truth? You can't handle the truth."

And the truth is that Cosmetic Dentistry, whether needed or wanted, is the Push Merchandise that if not for the "haircut" dentists had to take for treating patients with dental insurance would have likely been pushed to the sidelines.

CHAPTER TWO

Sex, Lies, & Tales from the Oral Cavity

2. What I Learned Selling Shoes for Pushing Smiles

The lessons in salesmanship that I got pushing shoes at my part-time graduate school job at Mister Jack's, a trendy women's boutique in the affluent suburbs of Short Hills, New Jersey, are the same ones that made me one of the most successful cosmetic dentists in the country.

If not for understanding the importance of showcasing the benefits of "life looking better when your feet do," I would have missed out on taking full advantage of my esthetic skills for enriching the lives of patients who not only put their mouths in my hands, but their faith and savings as well.

I figuratively if not literally took the presentation skills that earned me honorable mention in the Shoe Sales Hall of Fame out of the box and up a notch for selling Rodeo Drive smiles to all who followed the Yellow Brick Road to the very end. It was there in a small professional building—with two internists, two ear, nose, and throat specialists, no curtains, no tin man, no lion, and no scarecrow—that I applied the skills I'd learned selling high fashion women's footwear for becoming the World's Best Cosmetic Dentist. And to be crystal, my office WAS in fact on Yellow Brick Road, as was the challenge for new patients to find, given the souvenir appeal of the town's street sign, which all too often went "missing."

What started out as Mister Alan, practicing what Mister Jack instructed for "treating each and every customer as if they were a patient under my care," ended up as Doctor Alan a mere six years later. That fate would give me the opportunity to care for (and sell to) real patients had to be more than a coincidence.

That I didn't undergo the epiphany of how to successfully present treatment alternatives to patients until after my very first case presentation in practice was shot down is no coincidence either. After getting an initial "no," it struck me that I needed to reverse the equation and turn patients into customers. Customers are the ones who are more likely to take the friendly advice of someone "helping them" than patients are at believing what their dentist is telling them.

I was no longer opening my mouth to change feet, thanks to Mister Jack, right on the money about pushing pumps or bonding porcelain. I began to use what sold shoes for opening the mouths of my patients to exchange their smile for the new one I'd sold them on.

The word *doctor* in Latin translates to *teacher*.

Teach a salesman to sell a customer only what she comes in for, and he'll be lucky to make his weekly draw (the salary advance taken against commissions yet to be earned). Teach him how to change a customer's mind and sell her what makes him the most commission, and he'll never need to rely on luck again.

Necessity is more like being the Mother of Intervention (no disrespect to Frank Zappa or his Mothers of Invention) as anyone who has ever held a sales position where salary is based on a percentage of what you write up on the sales slip will tell you. And what's necessary is intervening, if you will, by inventing whatever it takes to steer a customer in the direction that nets the highest commission.

Salesmanship is synonymous with showmanship, whether in person, on the phone, web, Rodeo Drive, or as *The Wizard of Oz* demonstrated to movie audiences around the world, for selling trips down Yellow Brick Road, where all your wishes will come true.

The effective selling of elective cosmetic dentistry comes down to obeying the First Commandment of High Commissions: Thou

SHALT Bait and Switch.

Knowing what bait to use and when to switch it is the key that unlocks the door for any dentist to sell more cosmetic dentistry than he could ever imagine.

I learned to fish from The Master, picking up all the right lines for landing the biggest of fishes.

You will come away from *Confessions* knowing how NOT to take the bait to avoid getting hooked on a pricey treatment plan that you'll come to wish you never nibbled at.

One more thing…

Why not wait to bet your bottom dollar on any
recommended cosmetic treatment plan until
the sun comes out the day AFTER tomorrow.

That should give you enough time to finish the book.

3. Plaque, Smoke, and Mirrors

In the early stages of designing a new office, I spoke with a number of practice management consultants, each of whom had their own ideas on the "build-out" of my suite.

While they shared the belief that form follows function, each of them presented me with a different set of directions on the best route for getting there from their company's version of *Dentalquest* (like MapQuest except the destination is efficiency).

After studying each firm's proposal I called back the company whose plan made the most sense.

At our initial meeting in my current cramped private office, the more senior member of the two asked where my diplomas were. I indicated he needed only turn to the wall behind him to see college and dental school diplomas, a recently re-framed facsimile of my license to practice issued by the State, a certificate confirming my having passed both parts of the National Dental Board Examination, and the professionally framed plaque presented to me when inducted into Omicron Kappa Upsilon, the National Dental Honor Society.

Without turning, he commented something along the lines of "No, not those, the rest of them."

He quickly clarified his inquiry lest I feel insulted, explaining that according to his firm's statistics, as the number of plaques displayed on their clients' walls increased, so too did a proportionate rise in treatment acceptance.

His office plan budgeted space for a designated consultation room where all four walls would be decorated with an assortment of "floor-to-ceiling" plaques—a strategy based on a twelve-year history of recording approval rates for treatment accepted that was, no pun intended, "off the wall" for getting them.

Good walls may make for good neighbors, but plaque-covered walls make for even better case acceptance.

When I was a kid all I wanted for Christmas was my two front teeth.

When I went to dental school all I wanted was to graduate.

When I opened my practice all I wanted was patients.

And now that I was building my first new office, all I wanted was some assurance that the only fillings I'd have to worry about were the ones I'd be placing in my patients' mouths, not the ones I needed for filling my appointment book.

To that end, I was advised that "making a list and checking it twice" for enough plaques to fill my walls was the place to start if I wanted to see my "stocking" filled with patients.

In other words, I was to become my own Dental Claus.

The consultants wanted anything that had my name on it professionally framed for strategic placement at designated *hotspots* throughout the office. The hotspots in declining value of impact: behind the doctor's desk; floor to ceiling on the wall behind the doctor's desk; in consultation and treatment room walls at patient eye level; walls visible from the reception area; entry and exit hallways.

They presented me with a tricolor chart of each wall having highlighted "value" locations. There was little doubt as to their take on what's hot and what's not. The bathroom wall at seated eye level opposite the toilet was one, the wall above and behind the toilet another. I think you can figure out why.

The consultants referred to the plaque placement plan (PPP) as Window Dressing.

I couldn't have made this up if I tried.

I will be the first to admit, I AM curious about where my doctors did their training and what schools they graduated from, which is the main reason I put on my reading glasses to inspect the fine print of what's hanging on the office walls before he comes in.

Once upon a time I would have been overwhelmed and even intimidated to question the advice of any professional whose walls were, for lack of another description, overly credentialed.

Knowing what I now know, the times of my being impressed by the magnitude of the width and breadth of window dressing has been replaced by mild suspicion. I take no issue with any professional who is proud of his clinical appointments, diplomas, continuing education record, special recognition awards, or Dental Society memberships sharing proof of these accomplishments in any way he sees fit. Tastefully mounting these certificates on the office walls is a great way to educate patients on the extent of their doctor's training and experience, something that I admit to taking full advantage of.

What I take issue with is using smoke and mirrors to make any doctor appear more expert than he really is.

This would be no more than a premeditated, deceptive practice to gain an undeserved advantage for being taken more seriously than your reputation and credentials warrant. It's bad enough that practice management gurus recommend window dressing; what makes it worse is that it works, and even worse if it's already worked on you. It's no different than professional baseball players' use of PEDs to enhance their performance and put up Hall of Fame statistics that without 'roids' wouldn't be possible.

With a new office, new financing, and new worries, I decided to play it safe and took the consultant's advice.

I was given a list of professional organizations, many of whom I'd never heard of, with instructions to contact the ones he checked off to acquire their certificates of membership to cover some prime high-value wall space. He justified the application fees and the considerable framing cost as one of the best investments in getting case acceptance I'd ever make, not to mention its being tax-deductible and eligible for accelerated depreciation.

Unless patients routinely say yes to elective treatment in a cosmetic practice, there is no profit. And this is the fear that the consultants feed on to persuade dentists to comply.

The story below illustrates how dangerous "gift wrapping" can be.

At the end of the last day of a three-day implant course I took in New York City, all of the graduates (course participants) were given the opportunity to purchase an all-inclusive implant kit (surgical drills and an inventory of implants) with its own color-coded cookbook-like instruction manual to guide us through the entire procedure, start to finish. We were told by the implant company sales rep, as well as by the doctor who gave the course, that we could go back to our offices on Monday with complete confidence in putting what we learned to good use.

The idea of experience being the greatest teacher had become null and void.

This is a secondhand summary of what happened next after a fellow graduate returned to his office on Monday and hung his implant Wall of Shame. I say this because the number of documents he had framed from this single course was nothing less than shameful.

They were tastefully arranged in high-value locations, I might add, strategically placed, making them impossible to miss.

The patient in question was so impressed with the sheer volume of plaques throughout the rest of the office that she never put on her glasses to read the fine print. The assistant recalled how taken the patient had been with all of the honorable degrees, something that came out during the course of her deposition in the malpractice case.

She never had time to get a second opinion as the office called the very next day to inform her that today could be her lucky one because of a last minute opening in tomorrow's schedule; what turned out to be a not so lucky fast track to the start of her treatment plan. The dentist's deposition confirmed that the date of the patient's surgery was exactly two weeks from his first day of attendance at the "all-inclusive" three-day implant course.

He testified at trial on his own behalf that although this was the office's first implant case, there wasn't any negligence on his part that would have contributed to the failure of all eight blade implants. All eight of which prompted the Board of Registration in Dentistry to rule him ineligible to put anything harder than a toothbrush in a patient's mouth until their investigation was complete and his competency to practice dentistry determined. Actually, anything less than a ruling of incompetency for any dentist surgically placing eight implants on his very first case would be unthinkable as well as too late, because by then the damage would likely have already been done.

We may be naïve, but we're not stupid. We expect deception from a car salesman—actually a "car representative" because after you agree on price he takes the paperwork to his manager for approval, which you should live so long if it ever comes back accepted as is. If it does you're probably so grossly overpaying that they're afraid to risk any renegotiation for fear they'll lose the sale.

Not the case at a local Ford dealership when I tried to buy my daughter a car.

It wasn't until I was seated in the manager's private office and looked around that, suddenly, everything became clear. Not about the car, but about "high value." "Doctor," he said with a wall of floor-to-ceiling achievement awards behind his back, "what's it going to take for me to put you in this car TODAY?"

As I took in the window dressing, I experienced exactly what it's like to be sold on the other side of a plaque attack.

Dental practice management consultants are paid for giving good advice; theirs on the benefits of creating purposeful backdrops to gain case acceptance is one example.

What do you call good advice that teaches you how to manipulate others by obfuscating full and honest disclosure? Whatever you call it, there should be nothing with dental in it that's called for.

I'm for your cardiologist removing the plaque from your arterial walls and your hygienist the plaque on the enamel ones.

I had no reason to remove any of the plaques from mine, although I can't say the same for the dealership that I left to get a comparison quote from a competitor across town who, as it turns out, had what it took to put me in a new Mustang later that day.

CHAPTER THREE

Better Safe than Sorry

4. Kill As Few Patients as Possible

We, as your doctors, share a common goal that patients—regardless of ability to pay, refusal to pander to our egos, or failure to cooperate during treatment—deserve to come out of their dental appointments alive.

An American Airlines captain and all-American ski buddy puts it another way: Anything less than landing an aircraft on the center of the runway 100 percent of the time is inexcusable.

In fact veering off the runway for any reason from zero visibility to an approaching tsunami calls for a mandatory FAA investigation that can result in a loss of their flying license, even though the end result was a safe landing absent any passenger injuries.

The health care professional mantra to "do no harm" comes under The First Commandment of Patient Care: **Thou Shalt Not Kill Your Patient.** If there was a Second One it would be: **Please, Just Don't Let It Happen to One of Mine.**

That we could be called upon to save a patient does not come as a big surprise, considering that a significant part of our training in dental school overlaps the medical school curriculum on emergency treatment, which in many universities is the same for both dental and medical students. The intent is to prepare us to act swiftly and decisively in overcoming any life-threatening crisis should it occur on our watch.

We own the responsibility of keeping you alive from the time you enter the reception room until you physically leave the office. It's more than being a Good Samaritan; it's more like our license to practice holds us accountable for nothing less.

That your doctor IS adequately trained to save your life in the face of a medical emergency is something you might ordinarily never give a second thought to.

Think again.

While no one can predict if or when an "incident" will occur, your dentist needs, just like a Boy Scout, to *be prepared* to take swift remedial action during any medical emergency that arises, no ifs, ands, or buts about it.

It all starts with prevention—the reason I began every day's treatment with a meeting to review each patient's medical history.

You might be thinking that in the unlikely case of a life-threatening emergency, what better place to be than in your doctor's office, right?

Whether it's the right place or the wrong place depends not just on your doctor's training but on how well he's trained his staff for following an emergency protocol. Sometimes you get the answer only after its too late, which is why it's so important to insure it is before you begin treatment.

My oral surgery instructor in dental school liked to joke that when your life-saving emergency treatment isn't working, to drag the patient to the restroom, lock the door from the inside and shut it before instructing the receptionist to call 911.

I doubt that you find this amusing.

I've made a number of promises in my life that I've failed to deliver on, but I've never missed delivering on the one for exercising good judgment in making the right decisions for prolonging the life of any patient going through a medical emergency until the EMTs arrive.

Providing the right emergency care requires having an Emergency

Protocol in place, and the first place to start when you go back to your dentist is asking him to show you his. If you can't see it and read it, it doesn't exist. If it doesn't exist, it's a threat to your existence.

I initiated an ERP (Emergency Response Protocol) for everyone in the office to follow when the verbal alarm was given. The times I called for emergency drills to test our team's responsiveness under real-time conditions have proven to be the only ones that patients whose appointments ran late never complained about.

At no other time have more people expressed their gratitude for being inconvenienced. I'm not looking for your congratulations; I'm asking for your acceptance that if good health is not an inconvenience, it shouldn't be used as one for making sure that your dentist is prepared for whatever it takes…to keep you alive!

Why drills? Think grade school and consider that if there wasn't a plan in place that outlined what everyone had to do and where everyone had to go when the fire alarm sounded, it would have been chaos.

Speaking of fires, I had the local fire department come in once a year to have everyone who worked in the practice (part timers too) pass a CPR recertification exam. My colleagues thought it was overkill, no matter that it might prevent yours. I looked at it differently: If my staff doesn't know how to administer advanced life support, it could be MY funeral.

No matter how well your doctor prepares himself to handle a life-threatening emergency, it will never be enough when you consider the consequences of failing to keep a patient alive, never, ever enough if it's a member of your family.

There are lots of excuses your dentist can give for running late, but none for not needing or not having an emergency plan in place. There should be no excuse for letting him work on you if he doesn't or it could very well be YOUR funeral.

The only take-away from this grim reminder is that whatever can be done to keep it from being the one that gets posted on the obituary page is worth whatever embarrassment it may cause by taking the line from the film *Marathon Man* to ask "Is it safe?" before you open wide .

Emergency medicine taught in dental school, if my experience is the norm, is unquestionably very good. As for its ability to be retained, that's a different story. In the cosmic scheme of priorities during those four years of learning to be a dentist, the part about saving a patient's life is pretty much thought of as something only a RD (real doctor) has to be proficient in.

This should serve as an argument, a compelling one at that, for incorporating a recertification test in Emergency Treatment as a condition of each dentist's license renewal, what organized dentistry would without a doubt fight to the death, no pun intended.

The good news is that the majority of dentists can and do rise to the occasion when the emergency bell is rung.

The bad news is that there might be one who can't.

The emergency preparedness issue is one you should be asking your dentist about, but probably won't.

I maintain that NOT questioning your doctor's readiness to perform life-saving emergency treatment when it's YOU sitting in the chair is an ill-advised leap of faith that's not worth dying for.

At the very least, why not check to make sure that the restroom door can't be locked from the outside.

Better safe than sorry.

5. Murmur in Haste, Repent at Your Cardiologist's Leisure

Filling out today's comprehensive health questionnaires can be brutal. So many NO boxes for denying an endless list of diseases and conditions, many of which you've never heard of.

If you've been guilty of going into a "Just Say No" mode to anything you're too embarrassed to ask an explanation for, you've got lots of company. This is the path of least resistance for never having to write that "detailed summary in the space provided below" for each category answered with a yes.

The most curious exception in taking the road easiest traveled for speeding up the time it takes to complete the medical questionnaire as part of your New Patient Registration is the pause that's taken before signing off on a heart murmur.

For those who feel unsure about all of the NO boxes they didn't really know, it's a logical form of penance to admit to the "little one" you thought your physician mentioned after he finished listening to the message your heart was sending him through his stethoscope.

This is where a LHMONC box for a "Little Heart Murmur of No Consequence" could have prevented the YES that automatically opened Pandora's Box of unnecessary preventive medicine for more people than you would ever imagine.

The unfortunate thing is just like not being a little pregnant, admitting to having even a "little one" gets you treated like you have The Big One. This puts you into a high-risk category that leaves your dentist no choice but to comply with the policy set down by the American Heart Association to protect you from bacterial endocarditis, a potentially life-threatening bacterial infection.

It is this policy that mandates you take a preventive dose of an appropriate antibiotic prescribed by your dentist or physician before all dental treatment, cleanings too. A confession to anything "heart murmur" gets you an automatic life sentence of antibiotics, eligible for parole only when the American Heart Association changes its policy or when your cardiologist's letter gives you the alibi you need to reverse the verdict.

Everyone has heard some version of the horror tale of a patient who died after going to the dentist because of complications resulting from bacteria getting into his bloodstream that could have been prevented if only he had taken penicillin before his dental appointment.

There is no middle ground, "you say yes and I say no," as in NO, you are not going to be seen for your appointment unless you confirm that you have taken the prophylactic dose of antibiotic prescribed OR fool us with a quick comeback of a little white lie when you haven't.

The only comeback I have (if you fess up) is for asking that you do (come back) when you're medicated or contemplate the defense of an indefensible malpractice suit trying to explain my rationale for not prescribing a prophylactic antibiotic when a history of a heart murmur appears anywhere in the record.

No matter that you insist your physician told you it wasn't anything to worry about or offer to sign a waiver absolving me from liability; if you don't fill the prescription and take it as instructed, I'm not taking the chance that I could lose my license to practice by performing unprotected dentistry on you.

In June of 2007, the American Heart Association once again changed the guidelines on their recommendation for prophylactic antibiotics before dental visits. They also conceded that taking prophylactic antibiotics isn't exactly risk-free.

I've had patients develop upset stomachs, skin rashes, and episodic itching from long-term dentally prescribed antibiotics thanks to me. I've had to refer a number of drug sensitive patients to the hospital for antibiotics that could only be taken through an IV. And I've undoubtedly prescribed antibiotics to hundreds of patients who didn't need them, because I had no choice except to.

I can't help but think that if not for my following the guidelines, I'd have compromised fewer immune responses to infection on antibiotic overmedicated patients who might have overcome a serious disease, but didn't.

Not to be overlooked are the hundreds of patients I sent back to their family doctors for clarification on that LHMONC they recollected hearing from their physician, the hundreds of others I had to refer to a cardiologist for a definitive diagnosis to classify their heart murmur as either functional (calling for a preventive dose of an antibiotic before appointments) or nonfunctional (no medication required), not to mention the dozens of patients with heart murmurs that turned out to be "of consequence" that left my practice rather than conform with the American Heart Association's directive for taking antibiotics before every appointment.

I've had dozens of patients so dead set (no pun intended) against being "sentenced" to taking antibiotics before every appointment that they left my practice rather than comply.

There are an unthinkable number of patients who continue to pay a stiff price because they picked the wrong time to play it safe and hedge their bets in admitting to having "a little one."

IF YOU HAVE ANY DOUBTS about a heart murmur inconvenience aside, you need to consult with your physician before you "make your mark."

I remember from English class how the truth shall set you free, but should you tell a half truth about a heart murmur, be it a little one or one of no consequence, it's the truth, the whole truth, and nothing BUT the truth that while you may be free to go anywhere, you're not free to return for dental treatment (according to the American Heart Association guidelines for treating a patient with a heart murmur) until you pick up some "protection" at the drugstore.

6. Sleep Dentistry to Lose Sleep Over

Close your eyes, click your heels together three times, and think how Auntie Em's obituary notice would play in Kansas: After a courageous two-year battle with chronic nerve disease, Auntie to Dorothy, surrounded by her dental team, lost the fight to save an infected second molar as well as her life when she couldn't be revived by Doctor Drainbramage Scarecrow of The Oz Dental Group (it won't take much to figure out the names of his two other associates) who put her to sleep for a root canal.

Sleep is a convenient escape from the real or anticipated pain associated with dental treatment. It's also a state that can be conveniently and safely induced if you're at the right place for the right reasons and under the supervision of a qualified professional. Unfortunately there are some patients who arrive at the wrong place at the wrong time, which could lead to it being their last place—making it MY place to try to prevent it from ever happening to you.

If a sleep state can be induced to provide safe harbor from the dental experience, the only question might be why wouldn't all of us want to seek shelter there?

How great it would be to escape feeling needles in your mouth or blocking out the nauseating whine from the drill as it cuts away tooth structure?

The best part about sleep dentistry, aside from the rather obvious perk of not feeling anything, is it's over before you know it, with the added caveat that you don't remember a thing.

The worst part of sleep dentistry would be if you never wake up.

To that end, or better yet to avoid that end, it's absolutely essential that the credentials of the person putting you to sleep are beyond reproach.

Do not, I repeat, DO NOT agree to any form of sleep dentistry involving anything more than taking some pills or breathing a non-anesthesia mix of nitrous oxide and oxygen (that's analgesia) unless your dentist provides you with proof of having completed something more than a weekend course in conscious sedation. If it's a certificate for his attending a post-graduate course on "Putting Patients to Sleep for Profit," don't wait to smell the roses on your way out to the parking lot.

Exception taken if he brings in a certified anesthesiologist, what a fellow dentist and good friend offers at a separate and additional charge that's worth every penny.

As someone who took a "putting patients to sleep for dummies" short course, I warn you that allowing anyone who's taking this route to put you to sleep is a recipe for disaster.

My experience with such a short course took place at a NYC Continuing Education Center during my second year in practice. A check for $2,750 accompanying a completed registration form and a signed release absolving the presenter and the university from any liability was all that it took to be accepted.

Referring to our time together as a "mini residency" by the presenter, a practicing dentist and author of a book on sleep dentistry, he promised that after two days of lecture and one day for hands-on, practical experience performing the "art" (at his private office a mere five-minute cab ride away), we'd be ready to go back to the office on Monday and put patients to sleep for dental treatment.

The $2,750 turned out to be the best investment in post-graduate education I ever made bar none. In fact, if not for making it, I might have very well lost my license to practice or, even worse, been indicted for involuntary manslaughter.

I came away from that weekend experience thinking that any dentist who went back to the office on Monday and did anything more than hang the "diploma" we received at our Sunday afternoon graduation on the wall should be hung out to dry.

It wasn't until several months later that I felt ready to perform my first case, which also became my last.

It wasn't because anything bad happened; to the contrary, the patient did quite well and left under supervision (also dictated by law).

Unlike AC/DC's "Live Wire," it's not satisfaction guaranteed that if you get put to sleep by an inexperienced and uncertified conscious sedation dentist you live to regain consciousness and tell about it.

Allowing anyone to put you to sleep without the benefit of examining their credentials and seeing their statistics (all anesthesiologists have them) IS something to lose sleep over.

If you don't cancel your appointment for sleep dentistry before checking this out, it could very well be your last one.

CHAPTER FOUR

Why NO Means Not Yet

7. Earning His "A" Comes at Your Expense

Acceptance is what it's all about in Cosmetic Dentistry, and the WBCD understands this to a "T"!

If you read *The Scarlet Letter*, you know that the "A" Hester Prynne had to wear around her neck was punishment for having been found guilty of adultery, forced to endure daily ridicule whenever she appeared in public.

The "A" that stands for accountability is an undercover badge of honor worn by all cosmetic dentists who accept the responsibility for overcoming their patients' objections to recommended cosmetic treatment.

The WBCD's Credo: If at first you don't succeed, try; try again until you wear them out.

The acceptance success rate for elective cosmetic treatment is directly proportional to the case presentation skills of the dentist, the majority of whom will admit to being inadequately trained (if trained at all) in the art of salesmanship.

The avoidance of having to sell anything, even when it's for selling the truth about necessary health care, is what many of us thought we'd accomplished when we became doctors. The truth be told, the time for selling had only just begun.

This is an admirable character trait in a future son-in-law with a family business in the Fortune 500, but a recipe for disaster for any dentist who has invested his time, training, and capital learning how to perform cosmetic procedures but can't bring himself to sell life jackets on a sinking ship.

For those dentists who recognize that help is needed in the case presentation category, they need go no further in learning the tricks of the trade than spending time with an aluminum siding salesman. These "closers," as they are called, rarely meet a customer they can't sign, seal, and deliver on the dotted line of a contract.

Given the declining numbers of aluminum siding salesmen, it's easier to find a marketing course on how to sell cosmetic dentistry given by one of the many dynamic and motivational lecturers on the dental continuing education circuit.

There's no "semi" to the nonfiction report that you are hearing from one of these "dynamic, motivational, and accountability insistent lecturers" as we speak. There isn't a single one of my course attendees who isn't wearing the "A" around his neck, which for the record means he got his money's worth out of what he spent on tuition for learning how to earn yours.

In fact, if your dentist sold you on saying yes to a brighter, whiter, straighter, younger, sexier, more masculine, more feminine, or more powerful-looking new smile, you may very well have me to thank for it.

The secret behind this is really quite simple. An aspiring cosmetic dentist has to first convince himself how important it is for his patients to receive cosmetic treatment before he can convince them.

If the dentist plays his cards right, he will be successful in cultivating a relationship with you, which, when all is said and done, will result in YOU wanting to make HIM happy, and just like that, acceptance slips through your lips and winds up around his neck.

Any dentist wearing the "A" for accountability around his neck knows how hard it is to keep—something to keep in mind when trying to earn yours in "A"deptness for closing the door before he has time to get his foot in the way.

CHAPTER FIVE

Familiarity That Borders On Contempt

8. When it's Lip Service, Not Customer Service

Face it, you don't think about customer service until you don't get it. And it's not the being inconvenienced by the incompetence of others that exasperates us, it's their unapologetic indifference.

The gurus in the hospitality business proclaim that while making you feel welcome is crucial in turning you into a long-term customer; it's in turning lemons into lemonade where you really "make your bones." I call it "Recovery: Making It Right in the Speed of Light," which when executed flawlessly has the potential of winning a customer's (patient's) loyalty for life.

Dentists never imagined that they needed to be in the customer service business because historically, just showing up had always been enough to nourish a profitable practice. That was until the slow trickle they were hearing wasn't the water draining from the hygienist's cuspidor, but the rustle of patients' files being forwarded to the new generation of "touchy feely" competing professionals who were taking time not just for bonding teeth but for bonding with their patients.

This was culture shock for dentists who had only experienced practicing in the "good old days," or as some waxed nostalgic, The Golden Years of Dentistry, where the demand for services exceeded the numbers of those able to provide it.

In response to the growing demand for help to stop the bleeding, customer service seminars for dentists sprang up almost overnight, giving advice on how to keep current patients from going out the back door and getting new ones through the front.

For the first time dental schools were including Customer Service as part of their senior year curriculum and adding it to their continuing education programs for tuition-paying dentists.

"Institutes," in the broadest sense, were formed at faraway, usually warm and attractive places, offering training for the entire office and a take-home book of recipes for providing enough "knock your socks off" customer service to erase the frown lines of worry from your face.

Time for full disclosure: The *knock your socks off* thing was a natural for someone with such a successful shoe sales background (like me) to teach.

Customer service is more than an office sending you colorful reminder notes, more than asking you whom to thank for referring you to the office, and a whole lot more than routinely meeting your needs and saying thank you for paying your bill on time.

You get that when you renew your magazine subscriptions.

The not so new buzzword still works: hospitality.

It all comes down to respect, a lesson we should take from Rodney Dangerfield's introduction to the next chapter, to never allow a preferred guest to feel that they aren't getting any.

The profession learned the hard way that if you don't go the extra mile to make a patient feel important, they won't just leave without a desire to return—they may have left for the very last time. The majority of dentists do finally get it that unless they serve customer service the way you like it, you'll soon be ordering off someone else's menu.

That it took losing patients to make them aware of this isn't something that happened better late than never as much as something that never should have happened at all.

9. Crying Foul for Paying a Fair Fee

Pay for average, just don't settle for it

If you receive treatment that falls short of meeting the Standard of Care, you have a right to cry foul; in fact it wouldn't be right if you didn't.

If your fifty-five-minute appointment with the dental hygienist is cut in half with "sorry, she's running late," is the "I'm sorry" you get half the service at twice the price sufficient consolation for being treated (actually undertreated) unfairly?

That two I'm Sorry (s) doesn't equal an All Right needs no further explanation.

What will need further explanation is the groundless claim that no one in their right mind would make that's been driving my fellow dentists out of theirs ever since I made it: Any fee a dentist charges for treatment that doesn't far exceed the minimal standard of care is arguably unfair.

My familiarity no longer bordered on the contempt of my peers; checking my email confirmed that they were going well beyond that.

In this New Millennium of cosmetic dentistry, you SHOULD get more than what you pay for, not by accident but by design. If you consider the advancements that have been made in technology, materials, technique, and high-power magnification, all of which dentists literally have within arm's length, anything less than their exceeding your expectations would be 'uncivilized' (the word that's repeated in the TV commercials that's become synonymous with Charles Barkley, former professional basketball star.)

While many will disagree, it's time to rewrite the Standard of Care to bring it current and white out anything about "average."

Can you remember the last time you recommended an average movie to a friend?

How about the last time you ate an average meal, left the restaurant satisfied that you got what you paid for, and raved about the best average meal you've ever had?

Learning to tell if you've gotten above average dental treatment when it's not so obvious takes a little practice—practice that will be made perfect using my self-help clues.

That there is more to judging treatment than meets the eye is one reason why most patients don't have a clue unless someone gives it to them.

Determining what's fair and what's not is more often a matter of perception, taken right out of my "perception is reality" playbook, included in all of the courses I give to dentists.

- Who can't tell whether food is fair or foul just by smelling it?
- Who else but the dentist can tell whether your ceramic crown is the right shade just by comparing it to a color guide?
- And who among us doesn't know whether we're in pain or not?

How do you explain that the $2500 one dentist charges for a porcelain crown is just as fair a fee as the one another dentist charges $750 for?

How can you explain that the overwhelming majority of patients who knew they had paid more than three times the amount charged at another office never questioned the fairness of my fee?

It's when you believe you've gotten more than what you paid for, whatever you paid is worth every penny.

A sure fire way to improve your chances of getting the best is spelled out in my chapter on Insider Trading; it's a strategy for finding out the name of the best dentist around.

The same people who know the price of everything and the value of nothing can't tell the difference between fair fees from fees, fies, foes, or fums if they tried. (No disrespect to Jack of Beanstalk fame.)

You will not be one of them.

Whatever you pay for cosmetic treatment, regardless of whether you were talked into a service you didn't need; as long as the results exceed your expectations it's more than fair to me.

CHAPTER SIX

Respect, I Get No Respect At All[1]

IT'S BAD OUT THERE...

How bad?

When my fiancée told her mother I was a doctor, she wanted to know if I was a "real one"...or just a dentist.

That's how bad it is. I became a doctor only to find out I'm not a "real one." Respect, I get no respect at all.

I remember when I told my father I wanted to be a rock star; he convinced me that women worship doctors, so I left my band and went back to school. Now I find out that the only thing about doctors that women are praying for is being the recipient of his alimony checks.

By the time I figured that out, I'd been married and divorced three times. Now I'm sending out monthly checks in triplicate.

If that's not bad enough, my new girlfriend wouldn't believe I graduated from dental school until I showed her a copy of my diploma. When I did she threw it back in my face and told me she knows a fake when she sees one.

I get absolutely no respect at all.

Why, even my doctor doesn't give me any respect. His receptionist told me that he was running late when I checked in at 8:30 for my 9 AM appointment but promised that she'd get me in as soon as she could. After waiting three hours, I went up to the reception desk and

---

[1] Not only the quote attributed to the late great comedian Rodney Dangerfield, but the answer given by two-thirds of the patients polled in characterizing their relationship with their dentist.

told her I needed to reschedule because I had to get back to my office; As she picks up her intercom phone I'm told to sit for a minute while she sees what she can do.

Next thing I know she tells me is that the doctor finds me too demanding and suggests I go somewhere else for treatment. 'But I've been a patient for sixteen years!'

Sorry, she says, no exceptions.

So that you'll become the "exception" for never having to settle for lip service, read on and you'll learn how.

10. Getting Your Dentist's Undivided Attention

Undivided attention: Isn't that all anybody wants?

Once upon a time getting personal undivided attention at the dental office was guaranteed, an unavoidable perk for any patient receiving treatment at a "one-man show"—code in the profession for an office of one with a staff of none. This is how the term "solo practitioner" came to be: a doctor who practiced without assistants or assistance.

Those bygone days of giving patients their undivided attention were also the ones that didn't go by fast enough for a majority of dentists suffering chronic back and neck pain from standing on their feet all day long, stretching over seated patients while performing treatment. To this day, muscle relaxant addiction is one of the profession's best kept secrets.

How surprised would you be if personally greeted and seated by the dentist when you arrived for your appointment? Given the world that we live in, I'm betting that your surprise would turn to uneasiness once you realized that it was just the two of you alone in the office.

The solo practitioner's role in providing undivided attention to his patients came at a significant sacrifice. He could turn on the answering machine to get the phone, but there wasn't anyone he could turn to for cleaning up between patients, setting up the trays, writing in the records, pouring the impressions, sending cases to the lab, and that's just for starters.

He would, however, never have to worry about being characterized as a sexist for making the verbal gaffe of referring to any woman who worked in his office as "his girl" (as in "I'll have my girl get it") for the obvious reason that he was "the man,", and the only man for getting anything and everything for himself.

It seems logical that any dentist practicing without an assistant has a legitimate excuse for cutting back on the face time spent with each patient, given the overwhelming obstacles to overcome for finishing on time.

It may come as a surprise to learn that seldom was this the case.

The one-man show routinely finished each act on time, dismissing an audience who never received anything other than the doctor's complete undivided attention.

Today's dentist, proclaiming little choice but to delegate or die (physically and financially), has taken to the use of employing surrogates for many of the tasks he once performed—which will become even more if the changes proposed to modify the Dental Practice Act are put into law.

The staff has become a team, and the team has become the dentist's ticket to increased productivity by substituting his undivided attention with theirs in order to see even more patients. What's worse than your dentist spreading himself too thin is when you are adversely affected by his doing so.

You are not in the minority for thinking enough is enough when your treatment is repeatedly interrupted with "gently bite down on the gauze pad" as your dentist excuses himself to check another patient leaving you as a captive audience of one awaiting his return.

If you are satisfied to recline in the dental chair with a paralyzed jaw while your dentist practices Treatment Group Therapy, no matter that one of his assistants is sitting by your side to prevent you from feeling completely abandoned until he reappears, is up to you. When you've finally had enough, it's time to get his undivided attention with the words he can gently chew on: your unwillingness to share the time reserved for you so he can practice group therapy.

You have the right to ask for a somewhat monogamous relationship with your dentist, with the understanding that while a little "cheating" will be tolerated, there are limits to what you'll put up with for sharing his attention.

11. Isn't Your Time Valuable Too?

If your dental appointments routinely run on time, you might as well skip this chapter, count your lucky stars, and refrain from giving anyone the name of your dentist if you want them to stay that way.

If the possibility of there being a dentist who runs on time existed, the profession would have created an honorary designation such as a WBOTD (World's Best On-Time Dentist) to memorialize the accomplishment, one they haven't as of yet given the time of day to consider.

Do you ever wonder why dental offices rarely run on schedule?

One dentist I know used to tell his patients "It's because I still haven't made up for running late from my first day of practice".

I doubt you find this amusing.

Let me offer some insight. Each dentist has visions of grandeur when it comes to estimating the time it takes to complete a procedure from start to finish. Time management is not a strong suit most professionals know how to play, which isn't surprising since the model they learned on came with the magical safety net of the dental school clinical instructor to guarantee that everyone finished on time.

For example: The chair time it takes to complete a crown in a dental school clinic from start to finish averages four appointments, a total of eight to ten hours spread over four weeks, and that's if everything goes without a hitch.

In private practice the dental assistant brings the patient out to the receptionist to schedule the next appointment with a conversation that goes something like this: "Doctor Optimistic wants you to book an hour for a crown on Mrs. Never-Will He-In-a-Million-Years. Put her in for an hour and a half; it'll take him two."

[HELPFUL HINT: Getting either the first appointment in the morning or the first after lunch gives you the best chance of getting in and out on time for any doctor's visit.]

His time is valuable, and so is yours, but the only ones who actually do something about it are golf courses.

At most public and almost all private courses, golfers are told at the outset that their round will be put on the clock to make you aware that should you fall behind schedule (the time they have allotted for your round), a ranger (not the Lone one atop Silver but the other one who rides the golf course on a cart) will be checking to make sure that everyone in your foursome keeps up the proper pace. He'll warn you to speed it up if you're beginning to fall behind schedule to insure that all of the groups behind you finish their round on time.

Whether you practice on the golf course or the dental office, falling behind affects everyone. The reason professional golfers routinely finish on time versus dental professionals who seldom do is a result of enforcement.

Enforcement, what receptionists have failed to administer that Dental Rangers with the authority for lighting a match under anyone not running on schedule not only do but are legendary for doing to a fault.

What do you call a patient who informs the receptionist that he's not going to take it anymore for being inconvenienced when his dentist chronically runs late? I call him someone who understands that he isn't required to give the time of day to anyone who doesn't appreciate that his time is valuable too.

12. His Associate Doesn't Get You at "Hello"

If you've faithfully and promptly responded to each and every "please call and schedule an appointment" postcard from your dentist, you get two thumbs-up for following instructions, which you wouldn't need for telling your dentist where to put them. As in, what does he deserve for repaying your years of loyalty by handing you off to one of his associates, which he didn't think was necessary to inform you of until your next appointment?

What excuse could there be for a health care professional's lack of consideration in designating you for assignment without any explanation, prior notification, or the right of first refusal? That's actually a trick question, because it may never have occurred to him that he needed to answer to anyone but himself.

Imagine opening the front door on Prom Night and have your boyfriend's handpicked replacement hand you a corsage as he introduces himself as your date.

That's par for the professional course of taking liberties under the presumption that it's acceptable for one doctor to assign you to another. When it happens, it's usually at the last minute and not uncommonly goes something like this:

"Hi Mary, today's treatment will be performed by your new dentist, Dr. Ready or Not Here I Come, the associate Dr. I'm Through With You has personally selected to take over your treatment." .... As the dental assistant seats you for the appointment and your dentist's handpicked replacement enters the treatment room.

It all happens so fast that before you can open your mouth to object, you're being asked to open it wider for the injection, and just like that, the chance to "Just Say No" has passed as quickly as it took him to slip the needle past your lips.

The mouth is an intimate and private area, which means that no one (dentists included) can take the liberty of entering yours unless and until you give them permission.

This strictly women's issue is worth noting: The mouth and the vagina share a common biological basis as muco-cutaneous junctions. This fact is presented to make the point that having another dentist's hands going into your mouth is (or should be) as big a deal as having one of your obstetrician's associate's walk into the examining room after your legs are in the stirrups to inform you that he has been assigned to perform today's internal.

It would be bad bedside manner, not to mention unthinkable, for any OB/GYN practice to operate this way, as opposed to any number of dental practices operating as if nothing's unusual when a senior dentist assigns one of his patients to a new associate without giving them a proverbial heads-up.

No one can deny your right of first refusal, what many of those patients traded to an associate to whom they are first introduced while sitting in the dental chair might have blocked if they knew they could.

Remember that no doctor "gets you at hello" just by walking into the treatment room and introducing himself. If your newly assigned dentist tries it on you, I'd advise you to take off your patient drape, get up out of the chair, and lose him at good-bye.

Whoever said parting is such sweet sorrow, has never been properly introduced.

CHAPTER SEVEN

Veni, Vidi, Video

13. I Came, I Saw, Should I Be Convinced?

It may well fall under the category of "be careful what you wish for" if you "believe it because you see it" when you're seeing it through an intraoral camera. In fact if that's what convinced you to take it—"it" being your dentist's recommended treatment—you'll undoubtedly be more circumspect with your wishes.

First the good news: Thanks to the use of the intraoral camera for magnifying images inside the mouth, the "seeing it" aspect for both the dentist and the patient has never been better.

Now the bad news: No thanks to the tools in the intraoral camera's software, the manipulating of an image, as unthinkable as it might be, has never been easier.

The most telling intraoral pictures serve as exhibits to prove beyond a shadow of a doubt that what you are seeing simply can't be denied. If a thin fracture line in your tooth's dentin can be exponentially magnified to look like a crack along the floor of the Grand Canyon, you'll come off looking like a dummy if you expect a POF (plain old filling) to solve your problem.

If this isn't enough to move you to take immediate action, out comes a glossy color print—your dentist's selection off his takeout menu so you can share, with a designated other, what's worth more than the thousand words it would take to try to explain why a crown is the only thing that will fill the bill, nor should you fail to mention the check for $1,900 to pay it.

Should you remain unconvinced, the camera system has the capability for allowing your dentist to produce a personalized dental documentary that makes it "crystal clear" why you need to take immediate corrective attention. The quality and effectiveness of the DVDs I've personally choreographed might not sell ice cubes to Eskimos, but they worked well enough to convince nine out of ten patients who got one to schedule the treatment I recommended.

This could very well be an argument for Dentistry on Demand: A DBO (Dental Box Office) cable network that could make history by paying patients to view their own *Jaws*, which includes the details of your dentist's rescue.

I consider intraoral photography to be essential in the practice of dentistry. If used as intended there's no visual aid that can match it for patient education. When a patient sees an image on the screen at the same 2.5 – 4 power magnification that I do, there's no question about both of us being on the same page.

Should images be purposely and strategically manipulated, intraoral photography can't be matched for creating illusions in the same manner magicians distract their audience and trick the eyes into seeing the improbable. I can zoom in and make a small fracture line on your molar look like the San Andreas Fault faster than the time it took me to initial my last alimony check.

The majority of dentists use the intraoral camera to sell patients on treatment that's unquestionably necessary. What's uncalled for is that a small minority find it convenient for selling what isn't necessarily so.

It's akin to the wishful 'say it ain't so Joe'; a quote attributed to an anonymous little boy standing outside the courtroom during the Black Sox Scandal trial where Shoeless Joe Jackson, one of the members of the 1919 Chicago White Sox was attempting to defend himself against the allegations that he had participated in the conspiracy to fix the World Series.

You can come, you can see, and as reluctant as I am to inform you; if it's convincing you need, the dentist aiming the intraoral camera can provide all of the altered images he needs to sell you his treatment recommendation by convincing you that 'what you see, is what you get, and what you will be getting is 'indelible, accurate, and scientific, proof to make his point.

It's something to keep in mind when you look up at the monitor and see a larger than life intraoral image of the cracks in your molar. At the very least, it's worth asking for the thousand-word explanation in addition to the picture, because seeing isn't in the eyes of the beholder until he knows who *be holding* the camera!

If you ask yourself if you can put your faith in believing it when you see it?

Consider the case of Shoeless Joe's jury that saw through the manipulated images that were staged to fool them, that didn't.

Shoeless Joe was banished from baseball for one year.

Consider that if it's next to impossible to second guess dental images when there's no compelling reason why you should, the most likely outcome is to believe what you're being told followed by scheduling treatment.

I wish I could say it ain't so, but that would just be wishful thinking.

14. Mercury: Planet or Poison

Yes, there are dentists who actually believe that the mercury in your existing metal fillings is to blame for symptoms that range from forgetfulness and fatigue to a number of very serious and debilitating conditions.

While they have the right to speak their personal opinion, they have neither the scientific evidence nor an endorsement from any of the established dental associations to legitimize their claims. This hasn't stopped the few who disagree from making a one-sided case to patients to replace their metal mercury-containing fillings with nonmetal natural tooth color bonded composite.

I learned in graduate biostatistics that choosing the right mathematical premise to interpret your clinical data (medians, means, etc.) can support whatever scientific argument you intend to prove. This is the "putting of lipstick on a pig" by dressing up anecdotal[2] evidence in order to pass it off as fact.

An example would be a *can you believe it* recount of a person who, after having all of his mercury-silver fillings removed, throws away his crutches and begins to walk without any assistance.

Even if it did happen, without additional documentation to prove that similar results were obtained with other patients, it would be a stretch to claim that replacing "contaminated" fillings cured anything except the dentist's appointment book.

There is no shortage of compelling opinions from those in academia, entertainment, and health care arguing the health risks of allowing mercury fillings to remain in your mouth. If anything, they make for persuasive reading.

The erroneous claims that the ADA (and the dental establishment at large) is not doing what it should to protect the public by banning these potentially toxic restorations make for nothing more than sensational headlines to increase the readership for publications such as *The National Inquirer*, one of the many Journals for Expiring Minds

---

[2] Anecdotal—an unusual occurrence that results from an action that defies a scientifically supported explanation and any expectation it can be repeated.

available at supermarket checkout lines.

If you want to be entertained, go ahead and buy it; just don't buy the story.

If I had used this anecdotal rationale for proposing treatment, I could have very well lost my license to practice.

Such was the fate a dentist practicing in Michigan who zealously preached this concept to anyone who would listen.

Having personally attended one of his seminars I left feeling as if I had just come out of a Sunday morning revival meeting. He was so convincing that if I didn't know better, I would have come down to the podium and scheduled the exorcism of my poisonous fillings so that I could be saved.

Nothing, however, can save a dentist from exorcising the pains and penalties inflicted on him as a result of punitive action taken by a State Dental Board in taking away his license.

With religion, your beliefs are personal, and the decision to spread the word is yours and yours alone to make.

Practicing professionals, however, need to think more than twice before attempting to convert their patient population to accept treatment that runs counter to the gospel espoused by organized dentistry.

I DO FEEL AND CAN SCIENTIFICALLY SUPPORT my case for composite resin and why I abandoned placing metal fillings entirely. My decision is based on years of clinical experience, supported by fact, with nothing anecdotal about any of it.

Herein is my rationale for the preference of composite resin over metal amalgam:

1. It requires the reduction of less enamel and dentin when preparing a tooth for a filling, which in itself makes for a stronger tooth.
2. It decreases sensitivity after treatment when proper technique is used.
3. You get a more natural look when smiling or speaking by eliminating shiny metallic distractions.

4. It's less invasive and less costly to repair a broken filling because you are able to bond new composite to the existing one instead of having to completely replace it as you would for a metal filling.
5. You get a closer seal to tooth structure when you bond directly to the tooth. With no gap between the filling material and tooth structure (not so with metal), leakage is eliminated, new decay is minimized, and temperature change sensitivity is all but neutralized.

The caveat is that it costs more, takes longer to do, and requires a higher degree of clinical ability from the dentist. As long as all the criteria have been met, the resultant restoration has too many advantages for not making it the preferred filling of choice.

For many dentists, an overnight demand for replacing metal fillings would be more than they could ever hope for. It would be akin to holding a winning lottery ticket in their hand. The ADA, however, has not delivered the winning number (or opinion) for cashing anything, at least for now.

No more empty appointment time, an opportunity to provide more extensive and expensive alternatives to metal fillings without patient resistance, and a motivated population willing to take more immediate action when their health is at stake would be a dream that most dentists wouldn't want to wake up from.

That this dream lives on is what worries me about the decision to abandon metal fillings by a number of dentists using the persuasive argument that allowing mercury to remain in your mouth represents a health hazard. There are compelling arguments that can be made for convincing patients to have their current metal fillings replaced. That being said, in the absence of scientific evidence accepted by the Board of Registration in Dentistry in the state a dentist is licensed to practice in, using any of these arguments comes at the risk of having his privilege to practice taken away.

There's no excuse for any dental professional to offer up what can only be characterized as a collection of anecdotal evidence for predicting the harm of leaving metal fillings in the oral cavity or the health benefits gained by replacing them with a non-mercury-containing substitute.

If anyone uses this mercury scare tactic as the excuse for replacing your metal fillings it should sound off an alarm: the one that when heard calls for you to get up from the chair and excuse yourself on your way out though the reception room door

CHAPTER EIGHT

Is It Safe?

(It wasn't for Dustin Hoffman in the 1976 movie *The Marathon Man*.)

Is it safe? The most cited reason given for avoiding dental care since the film's release.

15. The Standard of Care: Am I Getting It?

Every dental student has to meet a standard number of requirements to graduate. He needs to score a passing grade on the National Board Examination that exceeds the standard before he can apply to take a required two- to four-day State Board Examination to demonstrate his technical proficiency for providing the standard of care before being granted a license for the privilege to practice.

This practice of dentistry is a privilege that is extended at the pleasure and under the watchful eye of each State Board of Registration in Dentistry (BORID). The Board is empowered to act with impunity in suspending or revoking a dentist's license to practice should an investigation (rising out of a patient complaint) determine that the clinically acceptable standard for treatment has not been satisfied. That the practice of dentistry is a privilege and not a right is why any letter from the Board marked PERSONAL is one that gets opened in private after consuming large amounts of antacids. The invitation to appear before the Board is an offer no dentist can refuse.

Malpractice insurance can't protect a dentist from suffering the wrath of the BORID. The only insurance a dentist has for performing his treatment conscientiously is attending to his patients' concerns, and if he's smart, "making it right at the speed of light" to make any complaint swim with the fishes.

The keeping of accurate records is absolutely essential in a professional's defense; anything less is a recipe for disaster that leaves the Board no choice except to make an adverse finding. Put this way, better to have bad records than no records at all.

Dentists do have a way to circumvent coming under the scrutiny of the BORID by instructing their malpractice insurance company to offer a financial settlement before the patient's complaint is taken any further. This liability insurance not only protects the dentist from having to pay court-awarded claims or negotiated settlements for damages out of his own pocket; it also keeps the details confidential. The companies issuing professional malpractice policies are responsible for dispensing oral hush money that makes the claims against their policy holders (dentists) go away, a smart business decision considering the grim alternative of a jury judgment for a significantly higher award.

Another barely audible best kept secret among dentists that most of us will admit to (in private) is that our best work was performed in the dental school clinic. If experience is the greatest teacher when it comes to clinical skills, how can that be? If practice doesn't make perfect, shouldn't it at the very least make it better? After all, if the filling that took two hours to complete in the dental school clinic only takes fifteen minutes in private practice, doesn't that indicate progress?

This 105-minute difference is not a result of the proficiency miraculously obtained upon graduation but the absence of a clinical instructor who approves treatment ONLY when it meets the dental school's standard. This standard is nothing more than the minimum requirement each dentist is expected to conform to for meeting the bar (without being supervised) after he earns his diploma, passes the National Dental Board Examinations, and is accorded the privilege of being issued a license to practice. I repeat the word "privilege" to make this important distinction: A dentist doesn't have a right to practice just because he has a license, nor does he have the legal legs to stand on for challenging the authority of his State Board of Dentistry's decision to revoke or suspend it. In other words, he is at their mercy, regardless of whether they dispense it rightly or wrongly.

In private practice the dentist is his own judge and jury; his conscience and his conscience alone is the sole guide for approving his treatment. Should a patient allege that he failed to meet the minimum standard of care, the dentist may have to answer to a different judge and jury as to: How in good conscience did you fail to recognize or correct the substandard result you produced?

What's puzzling is that if the quality of care provided in dental school, unlike fine wine, fail to improve over time, we need to ask: Why not?

Admit it, if it didn't hurt when he did it, looks and feels good after he completes it, doesn't break (at least not right away), and gets finished within the time scheduled, why would any patient doubt that they received the standard of care?

On the other hand, those of us who have the responsibility for providing it know exactly what it is, as we should. We also know when we haven't delivered it exactly as we could have for some of the excuses listed below that now you know too:

1. Running behind schedule and rushing steps
2. Failing to schedule enough time for a procedure
3. Lacking the experience to overcome a complication
4. Losing continuity to check other patients
5. Performing treatment that should have been referred to a specialist
6. Inability to get sufficient anesthesia to do the necessary drilling
7. Succumbing to the pressure of mediocrity to produce volume
8. Allowing a color match that's "close enough"
9. Using a double standard for services performed at reduced fees
10. Telling yourself that you'll redo it "next time," but never do

Running late is the dentist's #1 obstacle for meeting the standard of care. It's a pervasive factor in just about every complaint that the BORID is asked to investigate.

Your dentist is responsible for providing treatment that at the very least meets the standard of care. You deserve better than average; in fact, you should be getting what regularly exceeds it.

The good news is that this is pretty much a done deal from just about every fellow dentist I've met.

It only becomes a big deal if you wind up in the hands of the wrong fellow.

The Standard of Care: It's what's regulated by the BORID to insure that every patient gets quality of care without having to worry about it, except that you do.

If you do nothing else, do whatever it takes to find out if your treatment falls safely within the standard and "Just Do It" now.

16. Safe Dentistry, Safe Sex, and You

What IS a rubber dam?

1. Noun; a stretchable, uncomfortable to wear, tight-fitting intra-oral prophylactic to prevent contamination of the operating field

2. Plural: custom fit disposable sheets (not to be mistaken for Sheiks) that often come by the gross 3. alt. — what isolates the exposed tooth surfaces from being contaminated by the bacteria in the saliva 4. alt. — slang: dentistry's "one size fits all" condom. 5. alt. — a malpractice defense exhibit to document that "it wasn't me" who failed to take the necessary precautions while engaging in root canal therapy on a tooth that ultimately had to be extracted.

These square-shaped pieces of latex serve as a barrier in the true sense of the word to prevent the dentist from getting screwed by the plaintiff's lawyer, who would otherwise be all over him, assigning blame for his client's failed root canal.

No need to test for DNA, RNA, or TNA (if it even exists) to make a case for negligence.

Dentists are as damned when they don't as was a legendary actor for saying he didn't give one. Just as with the backlash from Clark Gable's classic *Gone With the Wind* utterance of not giving a damn, performing root canal therapy without placing one can be a nerve-racking (nerve-wrecking too) experience for any dentist appearing before the BORID who has the nerve to make excuses for not using one.

Every dentist—whether he graduates first or last in his class, a general practitioner or a specialist, charges an exorbitant fee or charges nothing, pleads temporary insanity due to a preoccupation with an acrimonious divorce (as if there is any other kind) is held to the same standard. If the facts that speak for themselves speak to the fact that no rubber dam was used, it will be damn near impossible for any dentist to escape liability IF root canal failure occurs within the statute of limitations.

Exceptions taken for modifying the standard technique by any dentist performing treatment is of no consequence, requires no explanation, and is no one's business but his own IF—and that's the game-changing IF—nothing goes wrong. The consequences arise when something does, and a patient decides to do something about it by either filing a complaint with the State Board of Dentistry or a lawsuit in civil court alleging negligence. Negligence that deviating from the standard use of a rubber dam has now become easier to prove.

There are times when you are asked to sign a consent form before treatment begins, but there isn't any consent you can give to absolve your dentist from liability for the adverse consequences that might result from refusing a rubber dam for root canal treatment.

There are millions of teeth that have been successfully treated with root canal therapy without the use of a rubber dam; I'm not talking about any of them. The one I'm talking about, which for you IS worth talking about, would be if it involves one of yours that fails.

For those dentists who are inclined to argue that it doesn't make a damn bit of difference whether you actually "give a dam" (literally and/or figuratively), take my advice and instruct your malpractice insurance company to use some of that oral hush money to settle the complaint out of court.

It's not always easy to place a rubber dam on a tooth, let alone keep it in place during the entire procedure: Clamps keep popping off, working x-rays are harder to take, it's more difficult for patients to swallow, it can become claustrophobic the longer it's kept on, and the final insult which isn't endured until after the anesthesia wears off is the trauma to the gum tissue from the metal clamp that holds the dam in place often severe enough to require pain medication..

All that said, one critical safety benefit far outweighs all of the detractors.

A rubber dam is the most effective way (actually the only one) to prevent any of those little sharp files that are used to clean and shape the root canals from accidentally being swallowed should one inadvertently slip out of the dentist's fingers. Surgery is often necessary to remove any of these that go down the wrong tube to wind up in one of your lungs.

I'll summarize with what a personal liability lawyer (an attorney who makes money by suing doctors) shared with me under condition of anonymity: As long as you put using a "rubber" in the record, whether you do or not, you're off the hook should one of your root canals fail and some "shamus" tries to pin it on you.

I'll be damned…so should you be for your next root canal.

17. Magnification: Leave Any Office without It

What doesn't look closer and clearer but not necessarily better with magnification?

That's a trick question, as anyone who has used binoculars to get a better look at someone they admired from afar only to be disappointed upon getting up close and personal: just like the reversal in grading the quality of care, which after further review is discovered to be inadequate.

The very first time a dentist views the operating field under high power magnification will be downright unsettling. The unsettlement comes from realizing that there is more than meets the eye when it comes to performing treatment that relies solely on the naked ones. The unsettling part is living with the knowledge that no matter how conscientious you thought you were, you had to have fallen short.

It didn't take more than "Just One Look"[3] for me to figure out that the treatment I could perform under high power magnification would leave the standard of care I had previously accepted in the dust.

The "seeing is believing" that we relied on to practice our profession in meeting, if not exceeding, the standard as defined by our State Board of Dentistry should by all rights come with an asterisk identifying the treatment performed under 20-20 vision to get you off the hook for missing what you wouldn't have with higher power magnification. A 20-20 defense for escaping liability might as well be double zero for the chances that any dentist will prevail when relying on it.

Think about the times you watched your dentist swiveling around in his chair for a better look at what he was working on, hoping that it was good enough. When you aren't seeing "good enough," what used to require an appointment with the optometrist now takes little more than a trip to your nearby CVS to pick out a pair of reading glasses.

The ability to see better will improve your reading ability, just like your dentist's magnification lenses should improve his performance. I don't know what it felt like the first time you put on reading glasses to

---

[3] Song by The Ronettes, a girl group of the sixties.

actually see the fine print without squinting, but I promise you that it couldn't even come close to the difference between working on teeth with or without magnifying lenses short of night and day.

Speaking of differences: There a big one between squinting to read a menu and squinting to remove the last bit of decay. It's one thing for taking off the hated anchovies overlooked in the fine print of your Caesar salad as opposed to taking off for the emergency room with a rapidly progressing swelling in your lower jaw that's making it hard to breathe.

What I am alluding to is that no matter what your dentist believes his 20-20 is showing him, he's kidding himself 24-7 when he thinks it's enough. He'll eventually find out, albeit too late, which is too bad for him; it's unlikely that you'll find out unless the consequences of his enough not being good enough require corrective care.

If you allow any dentist to work on you without the benefit of at least 2.5 power magnification, you have no one but yourself to blame.

I can't say whether it's negligence, oversight, or personal choice for any dentist who fails to come out of the dark ages to take advantage of today's magnification technology for treating patients who deserve nothing less than "cutting edge" before picking up a hand piece for doing any high-speed cutting on their patients' teeth.

The day I went from normal 20/20 vision to 3.5 power magnification completely changed the way I practiced, from that day forward and forever more. I credit this technology, as am I grateful to it, for giving me the good sense to understand the difference between good and good enough and the vision to make sure I wouldn't overlook it.

Practicing with magnification didn't make me faster, just better. Almost overnight the demands for more of my time to complete even the simplest of procedures wiped out all of the open time slots in my appointment book—to the extent that my receptionist had to start a waiting list for patients who were absolutely shocked upon finding out that they couldn't get in for six to eight weeks.

It wasn't because I was in such demand; to the contrary, it was a consequence of my needing more time for the treatment previously scheduled.

It's like opening Pandora's Box in that once your mind is opened to a new idea, it will never go back to its original dimension.

It wasn't just my mind, but my vision for seeing things in a way that I had never experienced before. I was now seeing my professional responsibility in a new light.

It's a different world under magnification, one where taking liberties with an American Express slogan pretty much sums it up: Don't open your mouth for dental treatment without it.

It's not complicated, the better your dentist sees the better….well, you know.

CHAPTER NINE

Finders Keepers, Referrers Weepers

IMAGINE THIS: Two dentists, Herman and George, had been practicing together for over fifty years and couldn't imagine what life would be like without coming to the office to practice the profession they loved. While fantasizing about the possibility of there being dentistry in Heaven, they made a pact that the one who died first would find a way to let the other one know.

It was a week later that George died.

A week after that Herman heard a disembodied voice coming from the clouds above: "Herman, its George. I've got some good news and some bad.

First the good: There's a Dental Heaven. Now for the bad: Remember that root canal specialist in our building you said you'd die first before referring even one of your patients to?"

If you mean the Endodontist down the hall who passed away last year, sure I do, but that's old news not bad news.

Well, he practices here.

So?

He just referred one of his patients to you and she's scheduled for this Friday.

18. Once You Find Them Never Let Them Go (to a Specialist)

To kill as few patients as possible is, without exception, the goal of every dentist from his first day of practice to his last.

The thought of losing a patient in the office and imagining the looks of horror etched on those seated in the reception room as they watch the paramedics' wheel a shroud-covered stretcher past them is enough to stop any dentist dead in his tracks, if you will.

A less disastrous, still painful, and far too commonly occurring loss is the one that strikes dentists exactly where it hurts.

It's The Center for Lost Income, a place for unearned treatment dollars lost as a result of referring a patient to a specialist in lieu of performing the work yourself.

The benefactors of The Center are the dental specialists: These are dentists who by virtue of the extra letters appearing after their names have a license to take as much treatment away from the general dentist as they can convince[4] him is not in the patient's best interest should they attempt it on their own.

In dental-speak it's called "referring to the man you use," code for a general dentist's sound clinical judgment for knowing when to hold 'em and knowing when to refer 'em; in preparation for avoiding that day when it will be the specialist's sound clinical judgment to determine whether the general dentist's 'specialty' treatment was in fact inadequate and is in fact to blame for a clinical failure. It's been intimated that a specialist's clinical judgment is 'colored' by their professional relationship with each local general dentist practicing in their zip code, referrers and non-referrers alike. Color me neutral on that.

The message is as clear as the one in *The Godfather*: Refer your specialty cases to me and I WILL get you off the hook; keep specialty treatment for yourself and you might be found swimming with the fishes.

---

[4] This is facilitated in many ways that run the gamut from specialists taking referring dentists to lunch, to becoming active in local district dental societies, or if all else fails to the unspoken insinuations that there could be "consequences" should a generalist's specialty treatment (usually root canals and complex restorative cases) fail and a disgruntled patient winds up looking for answers from an expert.

The physical act of a dentist sending a patient to a specialist is as easy as filling out a preprinted referral slip; the hard part is handing it over.

So while it's damned if he does or damned if he doesn't, it's a damned shame if your dentist convinces himself that he can satisfactorily perform your treatment and settles for anything less than a specialist's result.

Some will view the analogy between performing dental treatment and taking chances (also known as gambling) as inappropriate and unprofessional. Obviously, they haven't seen what I have.

I'll use the word "conundrum," because while most dentists hate to bet on games of chance, they don't connect the dots to realize that taking a chance is exactly what's taking place when they attempt anything outside their comfort zone of clinical expertise. In baseball, it's what happens when a batter without the good sense to lay off a bad pitch swings at three of them outside the strike zone and strikes out; in dentistry it's when your dentist "reaches" outside his. It's a bad bet, and what's even worse, the one who'll have to pay if it's a losing one is you.

We're not talking national security here, but it's a breach in the system when you're prevented from getting the highest level of protection by those best qualified to assure your safety.

Now I believe in good luck, but only in the context of paraphrasing the legendary financier Bernard Baruch's insightful quote about how luck sometimes opens the door, but the better luck belongs to the better players.

You obviously believe that your dentist is one of them and therefore would have no reason to question his decision to perform whatever procedure he schedules.

The enigmatic root of the problem is this: There are more than a few in my profession who will leave no stone unturned in performing as much of their patient's specialty treatment as they can schedule before they'd turn it over to allow them to come out from under to see a specialist.

I 'refer' to them as TURDS, The Uncomfortable Referring

Dentists who find that referring a patient to a specialist makes them uncomfortable.

The specialists aren't far behind in how they refer to them; 'those little shits'. I'm just repeating what I've heard.

When I asked several of my fellow general dentists who I suspected fit within this category to explain why they insist on "doing it all," there wasn't one who was willing to go on the record with an answer.

I assume they were all too uncomfortable to talk about it.

No doubt there is wiggle room to argue that performing specialty care for many general dentists represents nothing more than acceptable calculated risk based on their conscientious post-graduate continuing education and exemplary record of success. Patients of these talented doctors are at no more of a risk than they would be if treated by a specialist.

If you poll the current ranks of specialists, not all of them will be so generous in their acquiescence for accepting the possibility that any general dentist will get as good a result as they will. The record will show that for the most part they are 'right on the money': Specialists get better results almost all of the time.

I was taught in dental school that referring a patient to a specialist if I had any doubts about my ability to perform a procedure was a demonstration of sound clinical judgment. That I learned this from my specialist clinical instructors with a proverbial axe to grind is noted, as should you note that having taken this advice, has proven to be the best bet I've ever made in my patients' behalf. I say this based on my experience practicing with an endodontist, periodontist, pedodontist, and orthodontist in the Specialty Group Practice I founded.

If any general dentist thinks that he can walk into one room and perform a root canal, switch gears and perform periodontal surgery in the next, absorb the multiple interruptions of the hygienists wanting you to come in and check their patients, and still be productive and effective, he's 'got to be kidding'….himself!.

Okay, your dentist is fantastic, someone who does it all.

So I guess you could go ahead and "Just (let him) Do It." These RDs (Rare Doctors) are rare, but they are out there.

I offer one caveat if you are so inclined to remain in your dentist's office for the whole ball of wax: Convenience and cost savings are important, but not more important than getting your treatment from the most qualified professional.

It doesn't hurt to ask to be referred, which at the very least is the opening for a conversation while at the very worst, not asking might.

19. A Kickback for Referring a Patient?

I was attempting to take a quick snooze during lunch with both feet up on the desk in my private office when the receptionist appeared in the doorway to announce that the new orthodontist in town had stopped by and was asking for a minute of my time to introduce himself.

My 'have him come on down' response fit the bill considering that he was holding an invitation to spin the Dialing for Dollars Referral Wheel for any patients I'd be willing to send on down to him.

The essence of his message mirrored a familiar one from Ancient History:

He CAME to my office to present a novel but questionable referral award incentive;

He SAW that I was reluctant to get with the program;

He planned to CONQUER my objections for accepting $100 for everyone I referred to him regardless of whether they scheduled treatment.

Excuse me?

He argued that if it's legal for a lawyer to get a kickback (percentage of fees charged) when he refers a client to "a brother," where is there a problem?

I'm guessing that if you didn't already know this, you're probably wondering if it's your lawyer's policy, and not long after that to wonder if it's ever been applied to you.

Before you cast your vote as to whether this is unscrupulous, absurd, or unethical, you should know that it's strictly legal. It's a legitimate practice for one lawyer to ask for and accept a stipulated percentage of any subsequent fees charged for legal services by another lawyer to whom a client has been referred.

Surprised?

To add insult to injury, in addition to the likelihood that it winds up costing you more, your lawyer is not required to inform you about it unless you ask. And asking your lawyer is what you might want to do if only to satisfy your curiosity about whether he collected anything more than a thank-you note or a lunch if or when he'd referred you to another attorney.

As soon as he left the office, I put in a call to my lawyer to find out if he'd asked for or received, any fees resulting from the legal work the estate plan attorney he had sent me to may have performed.

His silence was not golden, which is why I referred myself to another law firm where the lawyer I met with informed me that while they don't make it a habit to ask for referral fees from other lawyers they send their clients to, it wasn't out of the question. When I told him of my habit of leaving any lawyer who would do so without first informing me, I received his assurance that this 'habit' would not apply to me.

As soon as I hung up the phone, I went into "executive session" to sort out what the orthodontist had proposed and what my new lawyer had inferred. Could I really remain impartial about whom I'd be recommending my patients to if I accepted his referral incentive?

I did some quick math: I refer about 200 patients a year, equally divided among three orthodontists who, for the most part, I select based on the office location that's easiest for parents to drive their kids to.

The "payback" from all three adds up to as many luncheon dates as I can find time for, an office that is guaranteed to be decorated by colorful rhododendron plants at Christmas, and any number of Harry and David fruit assortments that I'll receive throughout the year along with personal notes of appreciation for sending them my patients for orthodontic care.

Contrast that to 200 patients at $100 each or $20,000 per year for referring all of them to the one I'm guessing will sweeten the pot with as many lunches, plants, and fruit baskets that I ask for.

If feedback is the breakfast of champions, kickback must be a fine dining upgrade.

If you're curious about how I resolved my initial objections or whether I was unable to overcome them, contact me at theeclecticdentist@comcast.net and find out.

CHAPTER TEN

When the Cover-Up IS Office Policy

> "The truth? You can't handle the truth."
> —Jack Nicholson, actor

20. What If Your Dentist Is on PEDS[5]

Would the exposé on the use of steroids in professional baseball have been given the benefit of the doubt if the whistleblower had been a doctor?

For the record, if all it came down to was credentials in determining credibility, any professional ballplayers tell-all exposé on the widespread use of performance-enhancing drugs to boost their statistics and pad their paychecks would arguably have received less critical disdain than did Jose Canseco's if in addition to the record numbers of RBIs and HRs earned an M and a D came after their name. That in itself would have given justification for taking this controversy into 'extra innings' before calling the game.

In the absence of anything more compelling to support Jose's accusations than a recount of what he claims was witnessed firsthand in the locker room or snippets from conversations with his teammates, his 2005 *JUICED: Wild Times, Rampant 'Roids, Smash Hits, and How Baseball Got Big* was largely dismissed as little more than a sensational

---
[5] Performance-Enhancing Drugs

attempt to recapture the limelight from a baseball career that had long since left center stage.

He was possibly unjustly characterized as a self-promoting vindictive buffoon, an impression that not even his steroid repentance gave his critics any second thoughts about changing their minds

The sports fan's Forum for Expiring Minds, baseball talk radio, had an off-the-field -field day beating up his "giving up" the dirt on who did it, who hid it, and who he intimated was lying about it. No wonder it wasn't too long before we all got tired of it.

Those who initially had a hard time accepting the fact that highly regarded and successful "professionals" operating right in front of millions of admirers would resort to such things to become even MORE $ucce$$ful than they already were began to think twice.

In time, the early denials issued by several of the accused Hall of Fame eligible players were recanted. They begrudgingly admitted that the only cheek they had turned to steroid use was in reality the one they had been injecting the juice into.

And while there will be a number of asterisks placed in the record book to tarnish the accomplishments of those ball players who achieved them by using an advantage to gain an edge on their fellow ball players, consider this: There is NO asterisk that will ever be added to YOUR clinical record to set the record straight on the record number of porcelain laminate veneers your dentist sold you while operating under the influence of case presentation performance-enhancing steroids. All of which is beginning to sound more and more like a broken record.

To my knowledge security cameras are not standard operating equipment for recording cosmetic case presentations (although I allowed it in my consultation room subject to patient approval) to monitor the integrity of how cosmetically persuaded dentists entertain their fans with the pitch on how life will look better when they do' once they purchase a "ticket" for the express journey to their smile makeover.

Jose Canseco was never given credit for coming forward and breaking the code of silence to "tell it like it is." In a perfect world you don't kill the messenger, but in the real world when *The Truth Hurts* (title of Jose's upcoming fourth book), burying the body to destroy the evidence makes perfect sense.

In terms of CREDIBILITY, it's akin to the pot calling the kettle black when a steroid user becomes a steroid accuser.

In terms of CREDIBILITY, I readily admit to taking performance-enhancing action to boost my ability—not just to improve my case presentation skills, but for refining my clinical technique to gain the advantage of becoming increasingly proficient in how I perform treatment.

My drug of choice: continuing education, obtained outside of the office attending post-graduate courses that until now I've never admitted my addiction to.

What I will admit to is being an asterisk-free homerun hitter who makes no apology for everything I did off the field to make myself the best possible player in dental practice: To see that I did, you only need to check out my record.

And, unlike Roger Clemens, the memory-challenged former Red Sox Hall of Fame eligible pitcher, I'm not "disremembering" anything.

I'm also not calling anything black, just gray. I'm not blowing whistles on anybody; my purpose in refining your skills (like I refined mine) is so that you can tell if your dentist is on performance enhancers when he makes his pitch for recommending enhancements to your smile.

21. Fooling All the Patients All the Time

> **"A life spent making mistakes is more useful than a life doing nothing."**
> (Quote attributed to George Bernhard Shaw)

Dentists make mistakes, some of which we simply have to own.

The notion that we doctors would be excused for the error of our ways without any admission of guilt won't play in Peoria but does come into play on the practice field of health care. An example of this non-admission that rarely fools anyone comes in the form of a disclaimer attached to the settlement agreement negotiated by the doctor's malpractice liability carrier. The dentist admits to no liability for any damages caused to the patient and takes no responsibility for the same in exchange for a check made out to the plaintiff that whites out every allegation made.

It's called paying for fault that you don't have to admit to means paying in lieu of having to say you're sorry.

While the majority of dentists are inclined to give most people a break for having done them wrong in exchange for an apology, they are leery about putting themselves in a situation where a less than forgiving patient may not be so magnanimous.

Would you expect your dentist to inform you of anything that went wrong with your treatment before you leave the office?

The reality is that there are professionals (a number other than none should be reprehensible) who have developed an inclination for covering up their mistakes.

There isn't a dentist who hasn't made an error in judgment, with one possible exception. A New Jersey dentist attending one of my continuing education courses informed me at lunch that in his thirty five years of practice he has yet to make one mistake in judgment. (It must be something in the water, because that's only one better than the claim made by both of my New Jersey ex-wives in admitting that their only error in judgment was misjudging me)

If I may be candid, the chances of breaking bread with a dentist as perfect as my NJ course attendee is as likely as being served a grilled turkey rollup at The Last Supper.

If you have ever been a patient of Doctor I. M. Indenial, there's a reasonable chance that somewhere in your medical or dental treatment a complication occurred that won't ever see the light of day, let alone appear on your record.

Whether your record is an "oldie and a goodie" depends in large part on whether your dentist doctored the final cut or if there is an original recording that can speak for itself.

That's why I'm recommending you take my advice, the same given by every manager when they train a boxer, to protect yourself at all times, each and every time you enter the ring.

It's up to you to be on the lookout for any clues telegraphing that a massaging of the record may be in the offing, what my internist and good friend described as "rubbing out the potential pain that you caused by making sure there's no record of the wound," unlike the pain his ex inflicted on him that, for the record, returns when he sends out each month's alimony check.

What happened and what the record says happened is a perfect example of how it's possible the two twains shall never meet. With this in mind, I've put together an undercover surveillance checklist to improve your odds against getting fooled into believing that things are going exactly as planned when they most definitely aren't:

1. Watch the eyes of the dental assistant. If they stay in contact with the dentist for more than five seconds without smiling, something is up. Pay attention to the body language of the dentist. If he puts his drill down and looks back to the chart in the middle of the procedure, looks back inside your mouth, and then rechecks the record, it may be that he's been working on the wrong tooth, performing the wrong procedure, or maybe he's looking at the wrong chart. Don't act so surprised; this happens more often than you know.

2. If the dentist asks his dental assistant to have the receptionist reschedule his next patient, consider this as code for a complication that he hasn't yet found a way to resolve and/or doesn't have the confidence that he will anytime soon.
3. If you see the doctor or his dental assistant start to hyperventilate, consider yourself lucky if you get out alive.

The takeaway is this: The expectation of getting a full and accurate entry on your patient record is conditional, as in, under the condition that your dentist hasn't committed an inexcusable error in judgment that would only cause him pain, and I'm not talking in his quads, that he's unconditionally not willing to endure.

My friendly internist also tells me that just because something doesn't appear on the record that doesn't mean it didn't occur.

Superman's credo to pursue "truth, justice, and the American way" was something that as a Saturday morning cowboy-addicted serial-watching six-year-old sent chills down my spine each and every time I heard it. His superhuman example of playing by the book isn't anything like how the books have been cooked for recording a patient's mistreatment as anything other than well done.

So, remember to prepare yourself before you enter the Treatment Ring, and if you're lucky, you'll come out like the legendary fighter who grew up in the small town close to the one I did. Rocky Marciano, former Heavyweight Champion of the World from Brockton, Massachusetts was a man who knew enough about protecting himself to have never been defeated in a professional boxing match.

An accurate recording of the facts is something that a patient shouldn't have to fight for, except that you do. You expect to come out of the Treatment Ring with a decision of win, lose, or draw put into the record, but as it happens all too often in professional boxing, the outcome doesn't reflect what actually took place.

The act of fixing a decision is no different than a doctor whiting out whatever part of a patient's record he needs to for covering himself; what the ER nurse at our local hospital mirrored with her advice as I picked up the pen to make my entry in the hospital chart.

To err is human; for professionals who cover theirs up at your expense, it's inexcusable.

The last place you ever thought you'd be fooled has just become another place where when there's no record of the truth, it's because someone other than you can't handle it.

Jack didn't count on the fact that you can handle the truth; the fact is that it's hard to get a handle on it if it isn't put on the record.

22. Is Your Crown Made in China?

Dental laboratories came to be because dentists in private practice didn't want to take the time to make the crowns and bridges for their patients, which had been required of them in dental school. Granted, some practitioners do enjoy doing their own lab work, but the majority of graduates can't wait to send their cases to the man they use…as long as it's not them.

Time is money as well as a resource that dentists only have so much of.

This has become a business decision, a breakthrough of sorts, for a profession that has historically been inadequately schooled in finding alternative ways for reducing overhead to maximize profit.

The sudden increase in demand for their services resulted in a number of profit-obsessed dental laboratories farming out (outsourcing) some of the work in order to make more money, stay competitive on pricing, and get cases back to the dentist on schedule.

The consequence: Quality was no longer job one.

If you are open to another solution derived out of necessity being the mother of invention, it's not much of a stretch to see why I might be considered the Father of Dental Outsourcing.

I was a cash-strapped second-year student who set up a makeshift dental lab in his basement so I could moonlight as an unlicensed laboratory technician. No matter that my technical skills were a work in progress; if I didn't get enough work to make my rent, then technically I would be homeless.

I sent a letter of introduction to the half-dozen dentists located within a few miles of my apartment complex, offering to do their gold work at half the cost of what the commercial laboratories were charging. I figured I could do this and still turn a profit. Three dentists took the bait, all of whom, I might add, never expressed anything other than complete satisfaction with our business relationship.

This is how I operated: When I got a call, I'd make a pickup after I got back from dental school and confirm the date it needed to be completed.

Without exception, dentists don't like having to reschedule a patient because their lab needs more time, making the delivery date a priority.

Whenever the dentist's lab slip called for a tooth-colored veneer crown, it created big problems for me. I didn't know how to bake on the acrylic veneers, didn't have time to learn, and last but not least didn't own and couldn't afford to buy the special oven I'd need to do it.

I lucked out when I came across an unemployed oven-endowed lab tech in my apartment complex with lots of free time who I struck a deal with to outsource the veneering process for a flat rate of $10 per tooth. It got even better because he was on call whenever I needed him, guaranteeing that I could get cases back to my clients in record time.

I got all the credit for being able to complete veneer cases within seven days of the time I picked them up, as well the additional $22 I charged to bake on the acrylic veneer, yielding me an extra $12/unit profit.

The dentists loved it; the quick turnarounds and what had to be complete satisfaction with my work given that in my year and a half in the lab business I had yet to have a single case returned to be redone.

This is in itself amazing because no matter how unreadable (inaccurate) the impression and how mangled the bite record, there wasn't a single crown or bridge of the hundreds I made that didn't fit. I'll leave it up to your imagination to decide if I was really that good, or whether all of my dentists possessed a special talent for making it fit if it got past the lips.

I know I'm going out on a limb, but based on my personal experience there is no way you can have confidence in the quality of workmanship of any dental laboratory outsourced product unless you are given references. This is highly unlikely, given that no lab will volunteer that they are doing it, let alone who they are doing it with.

Unlike me, outsourcing to a technician who was a two minute walk away, the majority of professional dental laboratories simply don't have the time or resources to inspect that their outsourced laboratory meets the minimum standards, including infection control.

Look at it this way: If it takes over six weeks for your dentist to get your case back, it's possible that part of it was Made in China, something you won't see etched on the inside of your crown.

CHAPTER ELEVEN

Making a List, Checking It Twice...

23. "Give Me Five"...Things to Watch for

1. Your First Impressions of an Office

I know, Billy Joel sings about "getting it right the first time, that's the main thing," but don't go all in right off the bat. If life's experiences have taught you anything, it's worth repeating that beauty is only skin deep, something that those of us who married in haste are reminded of each time we make out our alimony check at leisure. There, I just repeated it.

Take, for example, an office with a cheerful receptionist who adoringly welcomes you versus another whose hygienist runs a half hour late and absolutely kills you (usually means a thorough job) when she cleans your teeth: If first impressions are the sole criteria for choosing between the two, it's a standoff.

Before you reserve a season ticket for The Greatest Show on Earth, take a look under the Big Top to make sure that the acts taking place meet the universal standards for infection control. Unlike what you get at the circus, your eyes need to be quicker than the hand so that nothing swept under the rug goes unnoticed.

First things first: You need to observe if the office is clean.

The constantly active reception room gets some leeway—not so for the treatment rooms located in the federally regulated zip code for patient care.

Making that list begins in the seated position on the dental chair for visible evidence that proper infection control has been performed PRIOR to the assistant seating you.

No matter how nicely you are treated before, during, and after your visit, an office that doesn't look, feel, or smell like its sanitary is a trick, not a treat, and should be avoided like an apple given to you by a stranger on Halloween.

2. This Will Only Hurt for a Minute

Your comfort should be the dentist's priority from start to finish.

Pain control is his responsibility, and any suggestion that it's not occurring because somehow you are overly sensitive is grounds for an immediate exit. That's E-X-I-T: Leave, as in get up, take off your patient drape, and spare yourself any further abuse. Reserve the "Just Do It" for buying yourself Nike sneakers, but unless you plan on putting your foot in your mouth, "Just Don't Take It" if it means having to endure pain.

You may not believe it, but believe it you should; there is always a way to make you completely comfortable. Like déjà vu all over again, it's worth repeating; there is ALWAYS a way to make you completely comfortable.

No matter that it takes more time or requires supplemental methods of pain control; you should never have to hurt for that promised one minute. Don't bother bringing in your Rolex to be repaired; it's not the watch that takes two hundred and forty seconds for his one minute that's the problem.

No one should tolerate being operated on in the presence of pain, that is, unless you actually prefer it. If that's the case this book won't take you where you need to go.

Abuse is a harsh word and I hesitate to even introduce it.

It's just that when a State of Dental Immunity to a patient's discomfort becomes secondary to the State of Finishing on Time, it's time for someone to stand up and proclaim, "I'm fed up and I'm not going to take it anymore!"

3. Make Sure He's a "Real Doctor"[6]

If there's a difference, here's what it should mean to you.

Even if you don't think so, Real Doctor rules apply when you go for dental treatment.

There has to be a complete medical and dental history review before any treatment can begin. Dentists need to know about your diseases, medications, previous surgeries, and a list of your physicians (Real Doctors) to contact at our discretion.

A heads-up for the guys: You don't have to list any of the online-obtained erectile dysfunction meds you keep in your night table unless you plan on taking one before your appointment.

For the gals: We don't need to know whether they are natural, silicone, or saline. You can keep this elective cosmetic enhancement to yourself.

In that we treat real patients; all dentists are prepared to handle real-time, life-threatening emergencies. For you to have any chance of surviving a sudden, unexpected medical crisis while you are having dental treatment, you better make sure there isn't any difference between what we'd do that any "real" doctor wouldn't. To that end, obtain reassurance that there is a crash cart with life-saving medications available; there is an emergency protocol in place that everyone in the office has practiced (to make perfect); and every staff member is not just certified in CPR but has been recertified within the past year.

If you don't go the extra mile beyond your first impressions, your lasting one could very well be from the stretcher the paramedics are wheeling you out through the reception room on.

If you're not asked real doctor health questions and your medical history isn't conscientiously reviewed by your dentist, there's a good chance that my ex-mother-in-law knew what she was talking about.

---

[6] What my ex-mother-in-law wanted to know when her daughter introduced me, "Or are you just a dentist?"

4. The Whisper You OVERHEAR that's UNHEARD of

Most of us are observant and usually pay attention to what the doctor is saying, although it's next to impossible to retain everything against the backdrop of so many distractions, our anxiety being a big one.

Which is why one of the most effective ways to get a point across, and one of the sneakiest best kept secrets for getting case acceptance, is letting a patient think that they are eavesdropping on a dentist's confidential comments to his assistant. This could be nothing more than a for-your-ears-only orchestration that you can't help but overhear. Let me emphasize the "could be" part, which FYI has never been and could never be anything I'd condone or have ever done. Sadly, I can't speak for those whose comments questioning the quality of another dentist's treatment are purposely whispered within your earshot, with no other purpose than to sell you on the urgency of correcting them.

The "sting" is obvious. It's the appeal of coming into inside information that you can use to your advantage. Isn't it a stroke of good luck to be sitting in the right chair at the right time to get the skinny on your past dental treatment?

I mean, if you overhear a whispered discussion about something that isn't done right and better be replaced before it becomes symptomatic knowing that a doctor would never go on record to criticize another, what more proof would you need to get started with the treatment recommended?

Most of the time whatever you hear in a dental office IS worth listening to, but as you'll come to learn, not all of the time for making the right decision as the case below illustrates.

5. You Came, You Saw, You Overheard , so Do You Schedule?

After all is said and done, there comes the time after you are presented with what's wrong for deciding whether now's the time to make it right is.

When I lecture dentists on how to get the maximum reward from their case presentations, I advise them to proceed as if each and every patient has come for their best and finest and shouldn't be offered anything less.

While most patients' needs can be satisfied with something other than what's optimally suggested, there is no excuse to present anything except what's ideal. There is no better investment than the one that benefits your oral health, and the last thing you want to discover is that your dentist only offers it to who he thinks can afford it.

Such was the case for a new patient in my practice who, after selecting a less-than-ideal although serviceable alternative, asked for reassurance that she wouldn't die if she waited to crown the rest of her back teeth.

Apparently she had overheard an aside from her former dentist (who died of a heart attack at the age forty eight) to his dental assistant of how worried he was about her inefficiency for chewing her food properly that if not corrected with crowns to rebuild the biting surfaces could very well result in a nutritional deficiency with far reaching consequences.

I admit I was intrigued, although taken aback, that any dentist might actually believe that placing crowns on all of a patient's back teeth (sixteen in all) could extend their life. Taken aback turned to taken by surprise when I couldn't find any mention about it in the copy of her complete clinical record that she had picked up from her now deceased former dentist.

I've decided to save this surprise for last, offered in the spirit of a lasting tribute to her former dentist's recommended treatment plan for doing a single crown a year in order to maximize her annual dental insurance benefits, although the possibility of her lasting long enough to schedule a single crown every year for the next thirteen (seven molars and six bicuspids) to complete her treatment plan was rather unlikely. At that rate, she would be one hundred and two years old when she made the appointment for the last one.

She Came: I examined her and offered my best and finest.

She Saw: I explained that she didn't have to wait thirteen years to see her treatment completed because I can do all thirteen at the same time and finish within two months.

She Scheduled: Incensed that the former dentist hadn't offered her the best and finest treatment available, which at age eighty-nine and one of the richest women in the world he'd had to have been a complete dummy to withhold.

Her words, not mine. My words were for expressing surprise at the check she left with the receptionist in advance of her scheduled appointment to begin treatment, drawn on the New York bank that bears her late husband's name.

I wasn't surprised that she left it, just confused that it was made out for $44,000 when her total treatment came to $33,000 until I read the memo at the right bottom of the check: that's $1000/year for the 11 you saved me.

I'm no dummy, I deposited her check. She got my best and finest, and I got her astonishment when I completed her treatment, start to finish, in less than six weeks. Everything turned out 'aces', and although she loved her new chewing power I'd made it clear at the outset that what she 'overheard' about extending her life by placing crowns on her back teeth is what I'd characterize as wishful thinking and not the benefit I based my diagnosis for treatment on.

She 'begged to differ'; right up until the day she turned one hundred and four, two days after what turned out to be her last visit with the hygienist.

24. The Dental Dummy "Cross Check"

"Cross check" are the captain's words you hear over the intercom notifying the flight attendants to perform a 'double check' before takeoff or landing.

It's not until they look 'one more once' to make sure that all seatbelts are fastened, all seats are in their upright position, and all bags are squashed under the seat in front of you before calling in a thumbs-up to the flight cabin and assume the 'position' in their jump seats facing you.

A cross check is what you too should do before letting the dental assistant put your dental chair in the reclining position.

While there are rather lengthy, detailed textbooks filled with lists of safety precautions, I've come up with a Dental Dummy Two Step that's good enough to satisfy Dental Traffic Control.

1. GLOVES — where, when, and for how long?

You should observe whether someone who is going to treat you washes their hands first before they put on a new pair of latex gloves. If they're already gloved when they enter the treatment room, you have no way of knowing if they have.

In this case seeing is the only key to believing, and I've seen patients refuse to remain in the dental chair until the dentist removes his gloves, washes his hands, and puts on a new pair, which won't happen if you're not watching for it. Take the time I visited a colleague (obviously not the World's Cleanest Dentist) who kept on a single pair of gloves the entire morning I spent with him, rewashing them before and after each patient without ever taking them off.

When I asked why, his response was something on the order of how "damn expensive" they are and how it's such a "hassle" to keep changing them over and over again.

Do you know what I call someone who acts that irresponsibly without any regard to the consequences?

A carrier of infection, and someone to avoid as you would Typhoon Mary.

It's better to speak up and risk hurting your dentist's feelings than putting yourself at risk.

2. UNIVERSAL PRECAUTIONS for Treatment Room Infection Control

No ifs, ands, or buts in determining through sight, smell, and sound that your treatment room has been sanitized.

I use the word "sanitize" because sterility (the standard for hospital operating rooms) is unrealistic for most dental treatment rooms as well as unnecessary.

Sanitizing is a time-consuming process that includes, but is not limited to, wiping down dental chairs with approved chemicals, hooking up replacement sterilized dental hand pieces, replacing the covers on all exposed handles on dental units, x-ray heads, and any equipment to be used during treatment, as well as providing pre-sterilized tray set-ups with dental instruments, burrs, cotton disposables, and whatever is anticipated for the procedure scheduled.

All of the above requirements must be met before you are brought into the treatment room.

A critical point I'd like to make is that in my experience it takes a minimum of five minutes after the previous patient leaves the chair to break a treatment room down and sanitize it properly before the next one is brought in and seated. Some offices, mine included, employ an assistant specifically for the breakdown and setup; worth their weight in gold because treatment room time is valuable, and the less time taken up for cleaning means more time for production.

That there IS a standard protocol for Infection Control that every dental office is required to comply with for guarding against and preventing the transmission of disease is of little consolation considering that it's rarely if ever enforced. That's about to undergo a reversal because it's time to revolt before 'the inmates take over the prison'.

If passengers on a WBCD airline flight don't get a cross check, shame on the captain; if you don't do my Dental Dummy Two Step before letting the dental assistant take your seat to the treatment altitude, you only have yourself to blame.

It's called self-enforcement when you're the one taking two steps and checking them twice before deciding whether to lean back and open your mouth for treatment or get up and take two steps out the door.

Ignorance isn't bliss; it can result in the transmission and/or contraction of any number of communicable diseases that you'd have to be a 'dummy' not to protect yourself from.

I'll take it a step further; don't rely on anyone but yourself to do a double check; don't think twice about standing up (out of the chair) when the results fall short; and don't give it a second thought if your red faced dental assistant does a 'double take' when you hand her a list of 'upgrades' that need to be satisfied before you're ready for 'takeoff'.

There is no room for compromise when it comes to your safety, that you're a passenger or a patient shouldn't make a difference. There's a saying about how the mind once exposed to a new idea can never return to its original dimension.

I hope that's the case for you.

CHAPTER TWELVE

———— *JP* ————

Insider Trading Without the Risk

25. Cashing in on Privileged Information

Every now and again, *Boston Magazine* publishes a seemingly special edition to identify Boston's Best Doctors; compiled by polling all of the doctors in the Greater Boston area for who they would go to if they had a health problem. The results are categorized by medical subspecialty of doctors' top doctors, which pretty much is the best endorsement any patient could ask for. After all, a doctor knows enough to take himself to the best, and given his access to inside information, who would know better than he but where to find it?

This is how doctors take advantage of privileged information to gain an edge, a professional's edge and a razor-sharp one at that!

A doctor's doctor is something to die for and just maybe a prescription to prevent you from doing that prematurely. It's also one that a longstanding patient of mine prescribed for herself soon after she got her hands on the name of my dentist, to whom she asked if I wouldn't mind sending a copy of her complete records.

She told me that it wasn't because of my fees ("you get what you pay for"), my staff ("the friendliest, most caring, and soon to be the most missed"), or that I hadn't routinely exceeded her expectations ("I have no complaints; in fact I really, really like and admire you"). It was because she so trusted my judgment that she knew I wouldn't go to anyone except the very best for my dental care, which is why she was willing to spend $48,000 for twenty-two porcelain crowns and a cosmetic makeover "like the one he must have done on you two years ago."

I can't say that I fault her rationale, because my dentist IS terrific, but had she done her own research, she would have discovered that she was already in the hands of the World's Best Cosmetic Dentist with little chance of finding anyone better.

You can't be prosecuted for trading yourself to your dentist's dentist no matter that you did so by taking advantage of privileged inside information.

It's gotten more difficult now that dentists are learning better ways of keeping the name of theirs top secret, but it's not impossible, not against the law, and fair game.

CHAPTER THIRTEEN

Foreplay That Puts a Smile on Your Face

26. Getting Lucky at the Dental Office

Do you know what the term "working girl" means?

I'm talking REALLY means?

You won't find it in Webster's Dictionary.

You won't find acknowledgement of the most distinguished ones in a Who's Who or read the names of the world record holders in Ripley's Believe It or Not. Don't bother to search through the Yellow Pages to locate one in your area, for that you need only to change colors and look in the red light district.

While curiosity may get the cat, all anyone needs to do to satisfy theirs is to ask any male over the age of eighteen the first thing that comes to mind when that's the answer they get to the icebreaker of " and what do you do" at the initial Close Encounter of the Third Kind.

For those who haven't gotten get it yet, "working girl" is code for someone in the oldest unlicensed profession selling a variety of personal services for fees that aren't likely to come under the supervision of a State Regulatory Agency unless they operate in the State of Nevada outside Las Vegas proper.

This profession, like dentistry, is always looking to attract new customers through the referral of existing ones who can't say enough (in public) about how well they were treated.

This could be how the phrase "it's been a business doing pleasure with you" came to be.

I've christened this dental aberration, Cosmetitution: the practice of wanton solicitation by a member of the dental team for gaining approval of as much cosmetic dental treatment as possible, applying as many tricks of the trade as is necessary to make it happen.

Don't be too hasty in jumping to the conclusion that the World's Best Cosmetic Dentist might be comparing the actions of a dentist to those of a pimp, which, although tempting, is what Charles Barkley would undoubtedly agree would be "uncivilized."

Consider what Cosmetic Dentistry IS and the concept will become clearer.

1. Cosmetic Dentistry IS marketed as being sexy.

The bill of goods to sell you a "Hollywood Smile" comes with the promise of increasing your sex appeal.

2. Cosmetic Dentistry IS an implied promise for opening closed doors.

What I'll imply is that when you allow circumstances to hold your common sense hostage, you won't have the good sense to resist DCPF (dental case presentation foreplay): the technique for brainwashing undecided cosmetic patients into believing that an upgrade of their face value courtesy of a smile makeover will so miraculously reshuffle the hand that Mother Nature in her perversity has dealt them that they can't resist reaching out for that 'key'.

3. Cosmetic Dentistry IS the seductive fantasy that life (yours) will look better when you do.

This overused clique is to convince you that once you pay for the ticket to get on the Cosmetic Express, a new and better life is yours as soon as the new you steps off.

If everything goes as planned, you'll come down with Cosmetic Immune Deficiency Syndrome or CIDS: a condition that paralyzes the immune system from resisting any further cosmetic treatment, one for which there is no cure, leaving those so afflicted with a lifetime habit of needing fixes that is all but addictive.

Once you suspect that some of these tricks of the trade are being used on you, the warning bells should go off before you lose the ability to prevent giving a Premature Acceptance to the cosmetic recommendations offered.

As the word gets out about how successful COSMETITUTION is in sealing the deal on scheduling more Appearance Dentistry, it won't be long before more dental offices use this to their advantage for sweet talking you into what you simply can't resist.

Hasn't that not always worked?

27. Cosmetic Immune Disease Syndrome (CIDS)

If you are a flower child of the new millennium, it's likely that you've been periodically tested for the potentially life-threatening but virtually preventable (when taking the necessary precautions) immunological opportunistic virus causing AIDS.

This highly publicized, debilitating autoimmune condition is most often transmitted by the passage of body fluids from a carrier testing positive for the disease to a partner who is exposed to it under the most personal of circumstances.

The aftermath of this not yet curable although somewhat containable condition brought about a paradigm shift of the "so never taking anyone at their word without seeing the written one (on a lab report)" generation's behavior. Spontaneity had been replaced by discretion for minimizing the chances of becoming infected.

And if that wasn't enough to worry about, out comes word of a bug that can be picked up in the normal course of making casual contact with your dentist's staff that destroys any resistance for saying no to cosmetic dentistry.

This condition comes through personal contact with a trained member of the dental team who knows the drill about leading you on until you no longer have the strength to resist taking a 'Cosmetic Course' (an exacting and usually long, drawn-out series of dental appointments to put the smile on your face that costs a lot more than the one you get from engaging in another course).

What can you, as a patient, do to protect yourself against the virus that gives you an itch that can only be satisfied by applying high doses of cosmetic dentistry?

Keep reading.

Knowledge is the key that opens the doors of reasonable doubt, whether to educate you about the dangers of engaging in unprotected sex or prevent you from jumping into every cosmetic treatment plan that's offered.

Thinking rationally is the antidote to counteract the effects of

CIDS. It's the self-inflicted dousing of cold water on your decision-making center for waking you up in time to overcome what your emotions are screaming for you to do. Unless you break the spell and conjure up some last-minute common sense, all is lost—not to mention a good chunk out of your wallet.

The thought of CIDS may not seem logical, but neither did AIDS.

They laughed at Columbus when he claimed the world was round, just as they balked at the research describing the role of baboons in spreading a disease that as we now know can be transmitted by humans and we know how that worked out. Could anyone have imagined that the remarkable myth-busting journey through *Boys in the Band* would only be part of the story? They didn't once the chapters had to be added for girls. There would be no safety for heterosexuals in a futuristic *Girl in the Dental Office* soap, a fictitious tale about how patients are seduced into accepting cosmetic dentistry by specially trained facilitators.

The bottom line is that you need some source of protection to prevent you from going all the way on a new smile to repel the spell of whoever is carrying the heater to melt your objectivity.

Success in cosmetic dentistry is directly proportional to the ability of dental assistants to put patients into a Cosmetic State of Mind. They are trained to do this at any of the "effective, reliable, and guaranteed income-producing seminars" given throughout the country: "Exceeding Expectations: May the WORK-force be with you" is the one I've given at dental meetings from Seattle to Boston.

I speak from the experience of having instructed dentists and their staffs to incorporate my presentation skills into their cosmetic case presentations to "achieve success beyond their wildest dreams," which I'm proud of and regret at the same time

Second thoughts ARE invariably wiser, which is what you'll need if you intend to remain CIDS free.

CHAPTER FOURTEEN

Leave No Smile Behind

28. A Prescription for Election Victory

I agree on the need to insure that no citizen in our country be denied medical treatment regardless of their ability to pay and without disqualification for any preexisting condition.

What I don't agree with is how to pay for everyone getting it when it comes at the expense of the rest of us.

We are being asked to act not just like Robin Hood in providing benefits for the poor at the expense of the rich, but barring Supreme Court intervention, guaranteeing blanket health care for everyone in between.

In a perfect world (or in an election year) it would be unthinkable not to extend a lifeline to help our fellow man get the medical care he needs just because his credit line has expired.

With that thought in mind, what comes next is not only logical but elementary, which even the legendary detective Sherlock Holmes wouldn't need much of a clue to figure out.

If we're not going to leave any man, woman, or child behind without giving them health care, how can we leave them behind with an unsightly smile?

Show me a man who says that good health can be sustained without taking a smile to the voting booth and I'll show you a losing candidate in their next bid for public office.

Why exempt the dental profession from taking an active role in improving the lot of our population? This has for too long been overlooked as illustrated by our medical policymakers' inaction to "get over it" and reclassify dental care as essential a service as it's medical counterpart, and dispel the current legislative designation of it being nothing more than an elective service.

I think that any candidate who fails to connect the dots to understand how creating smile lines will earn him support on the voting lines is following the recipe for a losing campaign.

I make this bold prediction: Whoever takes the position that the road to our citizens' health isn't complete without a trip to the dental office of their choice to obtain an All-American smile will be seen beaming his on CNN once the votes have been counted.

I have a good idea what the candidate who runs on this platform will be called: Mister President.

CHAPTER FIFTEEN

Encore, Anyone?

29. Curtain Calls are Vastly Overrated

There is no better tribute to a performer than an enthusiastic audience pleading for him to come back and give them more. That's what we play for—to hear those ego-stroking cries imploring a return for an encore.

It's what life is all about.

We want to feel the ground-shaking reverberation of stamping feet; to hear the decibel-breaking sound of clapping hands; and more than anything we want this to never end.

These are the "calls" I miss the most ever since I traded in my Fender guitar for a Midwest High Speed drill.

I didn't need Don McLean to remind me of "the day the music died", I got that on a daily basis from a patient audience who couldn't get out of their seats fast enough once my performance came to its scheduled end.

Not once have I ever been called back to 'please, oh won't you please do another tooth'?

My chances of that are as likely as being imposed upon to write yet even more chapters.

That's what I thought.

CHAPTER SIXTEEN

It's Not Complicated

30. It's the Ten Confessions not the Ten Commandments

Some confessions are harder to make than others, and it's not because I'm not man (or dentist) enough to step up and face the music for making my worst ill-conceived choices.

It's because I'm worried that the particulars of my acting like an ignoramus, heretofore admitted to and given absolution from in the privacy of the Confessional, might ever see the light of day, let alone the printed page.

That they have is a direct consequence of my repeated pattern of not looking before I leap, which if exercised with due diligence (or any diligence for that matter) could have spared me from embarrassing myself.

I've heard said, "Fool me once, shame on you; fool me twice, shame on me." But fool myself ten times and put it in print?

So much for what I should have known better not to do, which in the spirit of setting the record straight I'm about to admit to. I do this with the consolation of having been spared from settling up for any of these indiscretions pursuant to a most fortuitous coincidence. It seems that *Confessions of a Cosmetic Dentist* didn't go into publication until shortly after the statute of limitations had run out.

I may be naïve but I'm not stupid.

"A man should never be ashamed to own he has been wrong, which is but saying, in other words, he is wiser to-day than he was yesterday."
—Jonathan Swift, 1667–1745 "Thoughts on Various Subjects"

1. Jumping into the dental chair, I hastily covered myself with a drape, put a nitrous oxide/oxygen nosepiece over my nose, attempting to disguise myself as a patient to escape the vengeance of a presumably deranged (to say it mildly) gun-wielding intruder searching room to room for "that mother f…king sadist of a dentist who tortured my wife." It took me years to recover from the trauma of that incident that to this day, makes me think twice before seeing any walk-in 'looking for the dentist'.
2. I assured a very attractive local bookkeeper, who intimated that she did more than just balance the books on her weekend business trips to New York City, that there was no reason to worry about her bonded bridges coming loose. When told that she "used her mouth a lot" I loaded her up with samples of Biotene, a lubricating oral rinse, to prevent her throat from getting dry, that 'you don't have to spit out because it's perfectly safe to swallow.' Having inadvertently put my foot in my mouth and unable to open it fast enough to change feet, she asked if there was any way we could 'work it out' for having her bridges redone. I may be naïve, but I'm not stupid.
3. I didn't become aware of the typo on my fee estimate until after the patient's husband accepted my cosmetic treatment recommendation and asked if I expected to be paid the full fee in advance, our policy on all cosmetic cases. That's when I saw what should have been $16,500 next to Payment in Full Prior to Scheduling with an extra zero: $165,000. It didn't matter that I corrected it immediately and apologized for any misunderstanding, it was already too late. There was nothing I could say or do to spare him the embarrassment of looking stupid for

not only accepting that anything dental could cost this much, but for agreeing to pay it. I had talked myself out of $148,500; add an additional $16,500 to that because she never returned for treatment, nor need I mention did she ever return at all. I turned down a patient who agreed to a $165,000 smile makeover, I've never forgiven myself for being that stupid!

4. I was getting tired of being asked why my office was always so empty, too embarrassed to admit that having just graduated from dental school I didn't have many patients. Let me rephrase that, I hardly had any. I set about to change that impression by dressing up life-sized inflatable dummies to occupy the rest of my chronically vacant dental chairs so that any patient walking down the hall would think , *Wow, he MUST be good. All of his treatment rooms are full.* The deception was pulled off thanks to two life-sized mannequins purchased from an adults-only website guaranteeing delivery with "discreet" packaging. I fooled everyone except my UPS delivery man, who apparently was getting "patients" from the same website. Discretion—it's not only the better part of valor; it needs to get better for keeping doctor-patient confidentiality.

5. I was called on the carpet—mine actually—by an IRS agent conducting a field audit in my office who in the presence of my accountant admonished me for thinking that I was going to get away with taking a $550 deduction for women's lingerie purchased at The Fontainebleau Hotel in Miami Beach. Bad judgment aside, these were Christmas gifts I brought back for eleven of the twenty-something women in my office. I said I had nothing to hide, and challenged him to take any one of these young women aside and perform his own due diligence by asking them face to face before ruling on the authenticity of my claim. He didn't bite on the offer, electing to allow the deduction, although barely.

6. I completed a cosmetic makeover on a woman who died before returning to have all of her crowns permanently re-cemented. The bereaved husband demanded a full refund, claiming that her untimely passing prevented the treatment from being

'finalized'. I told my receptionist to convey my condolences, as well as to let him know that I'd gladly comply with his request in exchange for a signed release from the patient. (FYI: His now deceased wife had previously confided in me of her intent to leave him as soon as her treatment was completed.) My office manager seemed confused: "How on earth is he going to produce a signed release from his wife if she's dead?"

To which I replied, 'exactly'.

7. My receptionist added an emergency patient to our already full schedule, a distraught woman with a self-diagnosis of oral cancer who would "give anything if she could please be seen by the doctor today. When she got to the front desk to pay her bill, having just been given a clean bill of health and an assurance that she was cancer free, she went ballistic: I am absolutely outraged! Thirty-five dollars for him to take a quick look and tell me that everything is okay, you can't be serious!!

When apprised of this, I put a pair of gloves, some gauze pads, and a disposable dental mirror in a small baggie that I brought out to the front desk. I told the unappreciative woman to hand it over to any attendant at the drive-thru window at Burger King, stick out her tongue and ask him to take a quick look and see if his diagnosis is the same as mine.

She didn't see anything funny about this, nor did the State Board of Registration in Dentistry, to whom she saw fit to file a complaint. After taking a long look at the allegations as to my unprofessional behavior, the only thing they could have seen was how far over the line had I gone. I anxiously awaited the Board's disciplinary ruling, admonishing myself for losing my cool, and thinking the worst. I never received a notification from the Board, the patient never paid her bill, and while I never heard from her again it wasn't until almost ten years later under the most bizarre twist of circumstance when reaching up to pay the cashier at the drive-thru window at my local Burger King that we were 'reunited'.

8. A local physician complained that I hadn't given him the professional courtesy discount he was entitled to because after all he IS a doctor. I told him I forgot and apologized profusely for not having charged him more.
9. I interviewed a young woman in my private office who had answered our ad for an experienced chair-side dental assistant. When I asked her to identify any areas of weakness she might have, she smiled, leaned back, and crossing her legs so that I couldn't possibly miss the fact that she wasn't wearing panties replied 'it's probably because I'm too easy'.

    I told her that I couldn't work under that kind of pressure, fighting back those second thoughts that are invariably unwise before I changed my mind and hired her on the spot.
10. I've owned a number of fast cars; one of them was a fifteen-year-old twelve-cylinder Jaguar XKE 2+2 that a new patient, an Iranian carpet dealer, bragged wouldn't even come close to his new Mercedes 620 SEL. Not amused by my 'please, give me a break', he became so infuriated that he challenged me to a winner takes all race 'quarter mile, mile, first from zero to sixty, whatever you want'. When I called my lawyer for advice on how to word a binding agreement to compel the loser to transfer the title of his vehicle, his please give me a break was like déjà vu all over again. I got to keep the Jag, but that's just the half of it. Not only did I get a censure for unprofessional behavior, but since it's against the law to write an agreement for conducting an illegal act that I was caught living up to the letter of, I was issued a speeding ticket for doing 115 MPH in a 35 MPH zone. My automobile insurance premium almost doubled, not so much from the surcharge I was assessed upon notification of my "moving violation, most of it came as a result of adding a $129,000 slightly used car to my policy.

"What's done is done."
—William Shakespeare

CHAPTER SEVENTEEN

FOR DENTISTS ONLY

~This one's for you~

EXCUSE ME…HELLO?

TO ALL YOU NON-DENTISTS WHO COULDN'T CONTROL YOUR CURIOSITY ABOUT THE CONTENT IN THIS SECTION, CONGRATULATIONS:
YOU HAVE JUST TAKEN THE FIRST STEP TO HELPING YOURSELF. NO PATIENT SHOULD EVER TAKE WHAT A DOCTOR TELLS THEM AT FACE VALUE, PARTICULARLY WHEN THE FACE IS THEIRS.

THE NEXT STEP IS THE MOST CRITICAL ONE: PUTTING THE PERSPECTIVE GAINED FROM TAKING MY "CONFESSIONS" TO GOOD USE.

THE WBCD CAN ONLY HELP THOSE WHO HELP THEMSELVES,
SO PLEASE, HELP YOURSELF TO EVERYTHING YOU READ*.

*Except for the next 26 Lessons that only a Dentist will benefit from

EXPERIENCE IS THE NAME EVERYONE GIVES TO HIS MISTAKES* ...
(Oscar Wilde)

*Take the opportunity I'm giving you to learn from mine

1. Never become unglued, what a dental school classmate took to heart, actually to the backs of his earlobes with airplane glue so his ears wouldn't stick out like the legendary Disney elephant, Dumbo. Whenever you start getting nervous about completing a problematic procedure, thinking about the absurdity of gluing your ears to your head will put a smile on your face, result in an immediate thirty-point drop in your blood pressure, and, after taking a deep breath, lead to the solution of the problem you were stuck on.
2. Whenever an emergency patient with an out-of-state address complains of severe pain and states that anything you'd prescribe with codeine would give him a stomachache, the best thing you can do is ask an assistant to show him the door. Prescribing Dilaudid or Oxycontin to a possible drug abuser will not only get you hooked on answering excessive after-hours emergency calls for "something stronger" but a less-than-honorable mention on the watch list of suspected dealers monitored by your local police. More importantly, the preoccupation of dealing with their baseless after-hours emergency calls will make it harder to respond in a timely fashion to the authentic ones from patients who legitimately need you.
3. No matter how you are tempted by the convenience of taking a "quick one" (I'm talking a shower) after your early morning tennis game before you start to see patients, I'd advise passing on the option to install one in your private bathroom. One

day an assistant will innocently ask to use it on a day you've finished late because she won't have time to get back home to take one before she "meets a friend." If you feel guilty for keeping her past closing time and give in to her request, you have a good chance of being ruled guilty in a court of law for any number of indiscretions she could allege. And while you look for a criminal lawyer to defend you, you might as well check to see if his firm can handle your divorce, which is inevitable once your significant other decides to wash her hands of you as well. Who would believe that it's possible to watch everything you have go down the drain from a little shower? Don't put one in and you won't have to find out.

4. When your alarm company calls you on the inside line hours after everyone should have gone home to find out why they haven't got a closing, stop what you're doing and leave. Habitually working late to catch up on paperwork is a bad habit—made worse if the staff arrives the next day and finds you asleep at your desk. It's poor planning or an extremely convenient excuse for holding after-hours "consultations." How you take your poison is up to you, that is, unless your worst day in the office is better than your best day at home. In that case it will probably be your future ex offering to serve it up that should set off an alarm warning you to stay in the office and hope your alarm company is watching over you, too!

5. Perform periodic exams on women with a minimum of two of them in the room. In the New Millennium all dentists do oral cancer screening, now routine at every patient's appointment with their dental hygienist. Not so routine as I learned in my first year of practice when a young college co-ed pulled up her University of Massachusetts sweatshirt as soon as I entered the room, exposing bare breasts and clenching her eyes shut for "the dreaded cancer exam" that she wanted over as fast as possible. I couldn't get out of the room fast enough, getting a confused look from my hygienist who passed me on her way

in. The patient left abruptly without having her teeth cleaned, and I got a message from my receptionist shortly thereafter that her mother expected a call from me later that evening when her husband was home to answer to the outrageous examination protocol that resulted in having their daughter take off her sweatshirt for me to examine her breasts. Screening for anything on any woman without a female witness screening the process will take all the the spasmodic brilliance your lawyer can muster to keep your reputation intact for convincing a local court magistrate that there are insufficient grounds to send this case on to trial. I wouldn't put my hands on any patient without having an assistant present; I'll go so far as to advise you to avoid it like cancer.

6. Don't assume a mother is a mother until a son tells you she's his. I performed a new patient examination on a twenty-seven-year-old man with the same last name and address of an eighty-seven-year-old woman and current patient. When I told him how much I appreciated his mother referring him to my practice, he looked me straight in the eye and said: "My mother? You mean my wife." I looked him semi-straightly in the eye with "Sorry, I've confused you with someone else." This sixty-year difference makes a May-September union hardly worth a blink, except that in the blink of an eye because of a slip of the tongue he was gone.

7. When you can't come up with an explanation to satisfy a parent's outrage as to why the filling on her eight year old son's first molar has broken for the third time in two weeks, don't take it lying down, unless it's from your therapist's couch. Resigned, red-faced, and caught red-handed without any answer to mollify an angry parent who doubted my competency, the only thing left was to offer to refer her son to a children's specialist and pick up the bill, to which she agreed. Out of my relief came a lame attempt at making a joke as I filled out the referral slip about how 'maybe now you'll stop chewing on

rocks,' which as it turned out was far from lame. In fact, it was vindication when he answered something like 'not rocks silly, the little pebbles in my driveway!!!'

It's a good idea to keep some well quipped humor in your practice, because you never know when a wisecrack will come in handy for cracking a case, as well as saving your ass.

8. The holes in your schedule are ones that should be filled with R & R (Recharging and Relaxing), if you know what's good for you. That you don't is why your schedule is programmed for all work and no play, with nothing but worry to fill in any gaps. Since most dentists chronically run behind (if you are one how can you not agree) they're serving a life sentence for not practicing on time. Look at any open time not as a loss, but as the gift that you've been given for that well needed break to get your head together that might even help you figure out how to finish on time.

9. Wait until the end of the day to open all letters marked "Personal and Confidential" from the BORID (Board of Registration in Dentistry) with a piece of cellophane across the flap. There's not a dentist whose heart doesn't skip a beat when the receptionist hands him this letter or stops beating at all once he realizes that she's mistakenly opened it. What's worse is if she apologizes profusely, code for having read it and a virtual guarantee that everyone in the office 'won't leave home without (knowing) it'. A letter from the BORID usually means that a patient's complaint against you has been taken seriously, serious enough to warrant their further investigation. While you have no choice but to comply, that is if you value your license to practice dentistry, you do have a choice when to open it. Take my advice and postpone that until the day is over. Better to wait to ruin your day until it's almost over.

10. Refer as many of the lawyers in your practice to the dentist who is currently stealing (bad choice of words except they do when they can) your patients. It's time to own up to the fact that when one of your patients asks to have his records sent to

another dentist it's more that you lost them than it is their being drugged, taken at gunpoint, and held without ransom by one of the competition. Parting, however, can be such sweet sorrow, which you will experience when parting company with almost any Member of the Bar; who bar none cancels, misses, and reschedules more appointments than the quantity of shoes found in Imelda Marcos closet. This will go a long way towards encouraging your competition to discourage a request for a copy of their records from any patient in your practice. Res ipsa loquitor, in Latin legalese, translates to the facts speak for themselves. You don't need a lawyer to tell you what you already know, if your experience has been anything like mine.

11. Keep your knees together when you're seated in the treatment room. Sit-down four-handed dentistry with a trained auxiliary requires working in close contact—eye to eye, knee to knee—and keeping a close eye on where your knee rests, or rest assured you run the risk of being brought to yours should it inadvertently find its way between your assistant's thighs. Familiarity breeds more than contempt; it lays the groundwork for a lawsuit that can be brought with no more proof for alleging sexual impropriety than a 'she said'. As demonstrated in the "telling" testimony memorialized in a transcript of the deposition that opened the door to a six-figure settlement "without any admission of wrongdoing" by the dentist: Doctor that's a little more than my thigh, she reportedly said to his Sally, that's a lot more than my knee; which resulted in her jumping up and screaming.

12. Be a Painless Parker. Dr. Robert Parker was a grandfathered (not Board Certified) oral surgeon on Old Cape Cod whose name became synonymous with painless. There is no better way to achieve legendary status as a dentist than by putting your patients to sleep so they won't feel anything and better yet, if they can't remember it. For the majority of general dentists untrained, unwilling, and unable to administer general

anesthesia, the best chance at "making our bones" in the Painless Parker category is to give a shot (injection with a needle) that no one feels. If you want to be more than just a legend in your own mind, develop a technique like the one I used to gain the highest compliment of all: Doc, I didn't feel a thing, why you're even better than 'old painless'. I take issue with that because having known him as I did; I'll go on the record to proclaim that I've never met anyone better.

13. Keep your eye on the receptionist. This is the "voice" of your practice, which can either open the floodgates of new patients who after hearing it can't wait to come in or close down the stream so that only a trickle ever make it to your door.

14. Never put mirrors in your reception room. The last thing you want is for a patient to look into their partially paralyzed mouth that they'd like to ask the doctor about before they leave. Acquiescing to this request is tantamount to giving the captive audience in the reception room witnessing this enough of an excuse for rescheduling their appointments in anticipation of being further delayed from getting out on time.

    The first mirror looked into is historically one of the rear-view variety that's waiting for them as soon as they exit the office and get behind the wheel of their car. At that point, the odds favor driving home or going back to work rather than endure the inconvenience of retracing their steps back to the office.

    It's almost guaranteed that any office having a mirror in the reception area chronically runs late.

15. Collect all the show-and-tell models off your consultation room table, put them in a box, send them to the dental school of your choice, and take a tax deduction for donating educational aids to an institution of higher learning. Plastic reproductions of the anatomy might work for orthopedic surgeons, cardiologists, and possibly otolaryngologists. As for illustrating dentures and root canals, that'll work for giving your patients picture-perfect

excuses for canceling the appointments they were too embarrassed not to make.

16. It's never "nothing to worry about" until you get the results of a biopsy. The temptation to put a patient's mind at ease by relying on your skill, care, and judgment to make a diagnosis of WNL (within normal limits) for a suspicious tissue change, circumventing histological confirmation, is unskillful, un-careful, and ill advised, not to mention indefensible for excusing your bad judgment in misdiagnosing a malignant lesion.

    There is no such thing as inconveniencing a patient when it's necessary to rule out cancer, so if you plan on testifying at trial that it was something more than your intuition that determined a biopsy wasn't necessary, it better be good enough to convince the jury.

17. The only prescription pain pills you should keep in the office are the ones that another doctor has prescribed for you. Good news travels fast, which can only be bad news for you when the word gets out that a supply of "just what the dealer ordered" is available by prescription whenever his inventory is running low.

18. Never relieve anyone of their duties (as in firing them) without having your office manager in the room and a notepad in her hands. Overlook this and the relief of finally getting the courage to terminate an underachieving assistant will be short lived when she relieves you of the satisfaction of thinking that you've gotten away with it. "It" being what she alleged you proposed that would save her job. Two is definitely bad company (not to mention the name of a psychedelic 1980s party band) and while three is often a crowd, it's a lot better than a jury of eleven deliberating her word against yours.

19. Eliminate the five percent. Once I identified that most of my patient problems were coming from a small group of the rotten-to-the-core variety, I decided to spare myself from the certainty of future aggravation with the proactive action of giving them

(by certified mail) the required sixty-day notice to find another dentist who could better serve their needs, no explanation given. One hundred percent of the five percent didn't have any problem with this, nor did any of them call to find out why.

How do you like them apples?

20. When your patient has a headache, he may take aspirin. When he takes too much aspirin, he develops a tendency to bleed; if his bleeding can't be stopped he could die.

    If your patient tells you he takes aspirin for headaches, find out how often he has them or else it could be your head pounding should you have to call 911 and watch them wheel him out on a stretcher through your reception room door.

    The dentist in question never thought to ask a seemingly healthy patient with no history of bleeding who only took aspirin when she had a headache anything other than not to take any the week before her oral surgery appointment. As it turned out, she had been overmedicating herself with aspirin to get relief from what were reportedly as many as two dozen headaches a day. This was determined as the probable cause of the massive bleeding that could have been avoided if only the dentist had properly screened her by asking how often she was getting headaches. It's better late than never to learn the lesson that asking the right questions could save a patient's life; a lesson that came too late for the dentist who try as he might wasn't able to keep the patient alive while waiting for the EMTs to arrive.

    I'm confident that you won't repeat the mistake he did, which is the perfect segue to the next lesson.

21. Kill as few patients as possible. This is the best advice I have to give you for the obvious reason and some even better advice for the one that's not. Keeping them alive will avoid having to overmedicate yourself just to get through the day, what the dentist from the previous lesson needed for getting through his. So pay attention, because the life you save could very well be your own.

22. Never let them see you sweat. To err is human to forgive divine but to give a patient any indication of your desperation is not only an embarrassment, it's uncalled for. In fact it's the Original Sin of Dental Practice: the unprofessional error of losing face, for which there is no redemption from. When your chance of resolving a treatment complication falls between slim and none, ask the patient to rest her jaws by gently biting down on some gauze pads as you excuse yourself "to attend to an urgent matter." There is no greater urgency than for saving face, which is why you need to immediately take yours to a nearby private place to come up with a new plan before you return. Unfortunately, it's gotten harder to find that place now that the transition to digital radiology has all but eliminated the need for a Dark Room to develop x-ray film.

    When all else fails, return with a referral slip to a specialist and an excuse that's good enough to get you off the hook (for taking on more than you could handle), and you might come out smelling like a rose. It's not complicated, the less you sweat the better you smell.

23. When a patient tells you "I don't care what it costs; I want the best," its best that you wait for the check to clear before you begin treatment. Experience has taught me that whenever I'm told price is no object, it's not, largely because the patient has no intention of paying whatever I'm charging. Take my advice and accept the compliment that someone came to you because they wanted the best and who else but you did they think of, just don't compliment yourself until you've received payment in advance. You deserve to get paid for what you do, but if you don't, 'don't ask and don't tell' me that you didn't get precisely what you bargained for.

24. Hire happy people. Since you are Doc you get to pick who plays on your team. Pass on Grumpy, take Happy, and avoid behaving like Dopey for getting tricked into choosing someone for all the wrong reasons and none of the right ones. All it takes

is one bad apple to poison the office attitude, which is why you need to take as much time as you need to look through all of them until you find your Snow White.

25. Don't admit to errors in judgment, it's simply not worth it. Whenever you are overcome by the complexity of a case, remember the words that the NJ dentist attending one of my courses shared with me at lunch: "In my thirty-five years of clinical practice I've not made a single error in judgment." If you're that infallible, join him and my two NJ ex-wives as never having a reason to forgive yourself. Sometimes it's better to color the truth with denial, or so I've heard tell.

26. Don't be so quick to give a second opinion. Most of the married men I know get that from their wives without asking and pay for it when they follow it whether it's right or wrong. New patients get our second opinions all the time without having to ask, what most dentists don't realize until it's too late. Don't speak before you're asked , be careful not to make faces when you examine someone else's work, choose your words carefully when asked to give an opinion on former dentists, because one day the 'next' dentist will be asked about you.

EPILOGUE

The Final Confession

> **"Regrets, I have a few, but then again too few to mention."**
> —Frank Sinatra, "My Way"

Ask a dentist the treatment he performs that he gets the most satisfaction out of and more likely than not you'll hear the words Cosmetic Dentistry, the two words that for this, my Last and Final Confession, I've had a career long obsession with.

An obsession that was conceived quite accidentally at the Annual Meeting of the American Academy of Cosmetic Dentistry the first time I laid eyes on 'The Envision Computer Imaging System :the technological breakthrough that will forever change the practice of cosmetic dentistry as you know it". It wasn't too long into the visual tour, that it was about to change mine.

No sales pitch was necessary for convincing me how this 'cutting edge programming for putting a smile on every patient's face will put one on yours when they schedule it'. A special pricing discount, sweetened by an extra five days of training anytime during the first year for the convention price of $21,800 was all the incentive I needed. I don't know if anyone but me placed an order. All I do know is that I was one of the first dentists in my State to bring this technology into his practice, which with the one other that did make 'the two of us'.

It was lightning in a bottle. I wasn't just predicting a picture perfect future; I was bringing the future back to the present. No longer were patients worried that what they wished for wouldn't come true once I showed them it already had, not just on a TV screen, but on a side by side full color before and after photograph. The pictures were worth more than the thousands of words I no longer needed for asking you to 'picture it', when all you had to do was 'look at it'.

My ongoing preoccupation with this technology and the time I was taking away from my general practice attending post-graduate courses for staying on the cutting edge of all the latest esthetic techniques was taking its toll on my schedule with patients having to wait four to six weeks for an appointment.

Having arrived at that proverbial fork in the road, I took the path not just least traveled but never traveled and wound up where no dental practice had ever been. I created a Specialty Group Practice in Appearance Dentistry, identifying myself as general dentist concentrating his practice on esthetic improvement. This wasn't just different, in the small seaside vacation community I lived in it was virtually unheard of; but not once the local dentists got 'the news' and I began hearing about 'a snowballs chance in Hell' that I'd survive. It's what they knew for sure that just wasn't so.

What followed was unheard of success. I started receiving invitations to speak at dental meetings where dentists and their staffs were eager to learn my prescription for success, a Rx that would soon be filled in offices from Seattle to Boston.

I went on cable television to present half hour segments on the latest aspects of cosmetic dentistry; articles written by me began to appear in newspapers and professional publications; I became a founding member of the Northeast Chapter of a most prestigious national cosmetic academy as well as the initiator and founder of a distinctly different local Esthetics Group encouraging fellow practitioners to present their own patient cases and share ideas; I was getting calls from dentists asking to spend a day in my practice to sit in on case presentations to make theirs better. I've had the privilege of mentoring two remarkable dentists and former associates who emulate all that is the best and finest in providing patient care, not to mention their selfless contributions in honoring our profession. My good friend and the exceptionally gifted educator, motivator, and technologically driven cosmetic and implant practitioner who has taken my original practice to new heights will have to be patient at second best until after I'm gone before taking over as the World's Best Cosmetic Dentist. I'm in great shape, play a lot of tennis, and watch what I'm eating so he shouldn't plan on making his ascent anytime soon!

Imitation is the sincerest form of flattery, and flattered I am that my prescription for success has been refilled time and again.

Flattered, when your dentist's success in recommending cosmetic treatment resulted in your success for scheduling what you didn't think you needed that had he not drawn upon the presentation skills obtained following my prescription wouldn't have been wanted, agreed to, that once you did wouldn't consider turning back the hands of time to change your mind even if you could.

Regret, when a lot of what's being performed isn't as necessary for you as it is for the selfish reasons of the one recommending it.

Exercising reasonable doubt before acting on any doctor's recommendation is common sense, just as listening to those second thoughts that are invariably wiser before taking it.

It's much easier to be critical than correct
Benjamin Disraeli 1805-1881

AUTHOR'S NOTE

As a health care professional, breaking tradition to obfuscate 'the truth the whole truth and nothing but the truth' to write about cosmetic dentistry has been the best of times and the worst of times all rolled into one.

I confess to the little white lies, the massaging of the facts, the characterization of cosmetically persuaded practitioners as being obsessed with pushing Appearance Dentistry, the details of policy statements attributed to professional associations, nothing more than embellishments and half-truths to help move my story along.

That said, should the by-product of my semi-fictitious recollections give you pause to think twice before acting on a real time recommendation, take Bob Dylan's advice and 'don't think twice it's all right', because it probably is.

If you believe that truth can be stranger than fiction, you might be curious as to why I've gone to such great lengths (with semi-non-fiction) for making it harder to tell the difference. For one thing, I couldn't resist the temptation 'to tell it like it isn't', the best excuse for letting the reader's imagination dictate where perception ends and reality begins. And while tempted not to, this is the place to cover my rear by submitting a massive disclaimer for whatever I've described as being anything other than a fabrication.

If I'd opted to write a book of non-fiction it would have required doing my least favorite thing, verifying the details; don't waste your time trying to convince yourself that I have or that this is it.

If there's a World's Best Cosmetic Dentist, it's not me although that's not to say that I haven't tried. I doubt you'll find a dentist with WBCD after their name, exception accepted for it's presumptuous inclusion here. That doesn't mean that this unauthorized distinction hasn't been earned by any number of world class dentists whose patients' don't perceive them as anything less.

A good friend and 'world class' Cosmetic Dentist gave me this advice: If you decide to publish your story, better to say you made it up, better yet write it under an assumed name.

"When ideas fail, words come in handy".
Johann Wolfgang von Goethe 1749-1832
FAUST

DEFINITION OF TERMS

The Ones You Won't Find Anywhere but Here That Once You Read, You'll Know Why

A

AMALGAM: A combination of metals mixed with liquid mercury that has been used to fill teeth for over a century. The resultant mix has commonly been referred to as "silver fillings" whose safety has been upheld by the ADA despite concerns about potential mercury poisoning.

Dentists daring to speak out and question the safety of amalgams were warned to cease and desist lest they incur the wrath of organized dentistry and, in doing so, run the risk of having their licenses to practice suspended or even worse. Those "true believers" who refused to place them in their patients' mouths, recommending substitutes such as composite resin or gold, were looked upon as charlatans, accused of using the fear of mercury poisoning as a convenient excuse to replace their patients so-called contaminated fillings. There have been a number of instances where State Boards actually threatened to revoke a dentist's license to practice if he refused to abandon his stance, only one that I know of.

The moral victory, once the safety concerns of mercury-contaminated fillings received the long overdue scrutiny it deserved, came too late to compensate the losses incurred by those dentists who had the courage to stick to their guns.

Just like the pioneers of American history who traveled west to the new frontier, all they had to show for daring to cross traditional boundaries were the arrows sticking out of their backs, shot by those unwilling to explore the possibilities.

APPOINTMENT BOOK: The Book of Fiction that tells the fairy tale of a dental office that runs on time.

This is a Book that starts on time which even with the extra time his assistant tells the receptionist to schedule for will still never be enough.

No wonder patients complain "It's about time!" after being held hostage in the office for hours before they ever get seated.

It's a fable without the fairytale ending where: Once Upon a Time There Was a Dentist Who Never Ran on Time and Whose Patients Lived Unhappily Ever After.

While The Rolling Stones believe that "Time Is on My Side," patients are better served by telling their dentists that "time waits for no one" by not wasting any more of theirs waiting to be seated.

ASSISTED SUICIDE: A parallel universe where the patient has the right to choose how, when, or not to resolve what's causing their pain without anyone getting in their face telling them how to.

Extraction, root canal, or continued suffering are matters of personal choice that are not subject to being interfered with by pro-choice or pro-life proponents proclaiming they know what's best for you.

To my knowledge, there has not been a single report of a human chain of protestors demonstrating outside a dental office to prevent patients in pain from having a tooth removed that could be saved with a root canal. Pro-nerve is a dead issue—no one would have the nerve to stand in the way of anyone in severe dental pain to tell them that their options are limited.

ASSOCIATE: A dentist who works in your doctor's office who expects to "have you at hello" when you are put on his schedule. What consideration do you receive for your loyalty? You get the Two Step Double Talk through the lips of the dental assistant as you step into the treatment room and meet Doctor Ready or Not Here I Come, the associate of Doctor I'm Through With You "who will be taking good care of you from now on." This should get you to thinking that while membership does have its privileges, yours didn't come with a right of first refusal.

ATTITUDINOSCLEROSIS: The hardening of the attitudes that develop among dental staff who, unhappy with their jobs, their pay, the people they work with, or any combination thereof, make life miserable for everyone around them. This staff-borne infection is highly contagious and easily transmitted to fellow coworkers who haven't developed a resistance to this undermining virus. In the absence of a cure, all that can be done is to quarantine those infected and never let them return.

B

BILLS: The monthly printed statements of treatment charges accompanied by a self-addressed envelope that most likely never returns with any payment, let alone "the payment in full due upon receipt" asked for.

The dental practices who haven't yet figured out that the only ones who benefit from bills are ducks will likely come to that conclusion once four billing cycles have passed with nary a word ever being heard about paying them.

BORID: Short for the Board of Registration in Dentistry, a state regulating agency that wields autonomous power over a dentist's license to practice. In that licensure is a privilege and not a right, dentists have little recourse for overturning any punitive action taken against them.

The chances are that a letter from the BORID marked "personal" with a cellophane strip placed across the envelope flap contains an invitation to answer a patient's complaint made against you that the Board deems sufficient to begin an investigation.

Having personally survived several, all of which resulted in complete vindication, I admit that at no other times in my life have I lost more sleep or consumed more antacids.

BLEACHING: The Clorox-like action on discolored and stained teeth that turns them whiter and brighter with less effort than it takes to clean your soiled laundry. And while it costs more than the Laundromat, takes longer than your standard load, and requires that the attendant be a dentist, it's still a bargain and the best ground floor cosmetic entry point to rejuvenate a life that will look brighter once your front teeth are made whiter. You Can Never Be Too Rich, Too Thin, Or Have Teeth Too White is more than a patient wish list; it's the title of a continuing education course I've given to dentists across the country who have never made more for doing nothing more than taking my advice on how to sell tooth bleaching to their patients.

BONDING WAND: The business end of Cosmetic Dentistry's most significant equipment discovery since the high-speed hand piece replaced the foot-pedal-driven drill.

The white light wavelength emitted transforms soft and malleable natural tooth-colored composite resin placed in the prepared filling cavity into a hard and rigid state that's sufficiently durable for indefinitely withstanding the biting forces without breaking.

A process that pharmaceutical companies have been conducting parallel secret clinical trials on in hopes of identifying the "right light" that would give the same end result, in a manner of speaking, for treating ED (erectile dysfunction).

If you take a "hard" look at the benefits of turning on a switch for turning on the patient as opposed to waiting for a pill to take effect, the decision on allocating the necessary funding for recruiting additional male subjects to continue clinical trials would be a no brainer. The envisioned advertising campaign promises to be a winner: When the time is right, you'll never have to worry about anything more than simply turning on the switch and letting your love life begin.

BONDODONTIST: The putdown that many in the profession use in demeaning fellow dentists who call themselves Bonding Specialists. A term that, rumor has it, came out of the mouth of a plumber's helper who, having read up on how resin gets hard and sticks to teeth during the bonding process "when you shine some kind of flashlight on it," asked his dentist if he could have his corroded-looking fillings replaced with "BONDOS."

C

CIDS (Cosmetic Immune Deficiency Syndrome): The inability of the body's defense system to fight off any recommendation for cosmetic dentistry. Research is ongoing, and while the hopes of developing a vaccine anytime soon are slim, a number of complete and sudden remissions have been reported. These cures have occurred in the presence of a Greenback

Deficiency carried by patients who in each case didn't have enough of them to pay for treatment. This lack of fee for service is the only universal remedy currently available to combat the spread of this disease.

COBRA (Continuation of health care benefits that would otherwise be terminated): Not the poisonous snake found in India, but nonetheless something with the potential of taking a serious bite out of your wallet. I'm referring to the limited period of time that your health insurance coverage is allowed to continue between jobs, as long as you keep the payments previously paid for by your former employer current.

Rodney Dangerfield once referred to Shakespeare's "Ah life, where IS thy sting" in one of his comedy routines. If you're wondering where it is, just ask anyone paying for COBRA. They should know.

CODE BLUE: Heard in most hospitals or doctors' offices, code blue is the universal call to anyone within earshot for immediate assistance in dealing with a life-threatening emergency. Dentists, seldom called upon to deal with such crises, are too often guilty of delaying a call for help. (This delay is no great surprise given that most of them have never once practiced an office emergency drill.)

When they finally do (call for help), it's often too late for anything other than taking my oral surgery instructor's advice for getting a hand in dragging the patient into the bathroom and locking them inside before having the receptionist call 911.

COMPUTER IMAGING: With a software program that allows the operator to make changes in a patient's dental appearance, a coming attraction of their projected re-mastered smile is created for viewing in living color on a TV screen. First used in beauty salons to see how different hairstyles and hair coloring would look on their clients, computer imaging is taken up a notch to sell patients on buying the ticket for their Hollywood smile right after they are "blown away" by the sneak preview.

COSMETITUTION: Taken from the oldest profession that cosmetic dentistry has drawn upon to provide dental assistants with some professional tricks of the trade for wearing down a patient's resistance to get a YES to recommended treatment. It should come as no surprise that payment in advance before either of these professional services is performed is pretty much standard operating policy.

COSMONYMPHOMANIAC: A patient who can't ever get enough cosmetic treatment and, never satisfied, always returns for more.

CROSS CHECK: A checklist that flight attendants are required to run through prior to takeoff and landing that the one every patient should check off as they take their seat in a dental chair should be modeled after. You need to do a cross check to be certain that all of the necessary safety precautions for infection control that meet the standard of care have been taken. While both the FAA and the ADA have established safety requirements to protect their customers (passengers and patients), the only way to make sure they've been met is with a double check.

Based on my personal observation in visiting dental offices across the country, there may be less risk in flying than there is in getting dental treatment.

CUSTOMER SERVICE: The attention you expect from everyone in the dental office to make your appointment one to remember. That you even remember the words "customer service" is enough to remind you that you haven't gotten any. Most patients never fuss or complain about having settled for lip service because that wouldn't be nice. Instead they just put their words together to discreetly, but nicely, blow the office off as payback for the disservice endured. These patients aren't only nice; they're ones who never return.

D

DARK ROOM: A small light-free pantry-sized room in every dental office reserved for developing x-rays that became obsolete when digital radiography produced the same images onto a computer screen in the full light of day. The transformation of this cubicle to a supply closet was an even darker day for dentists who no longer had a "safe house" to compose themselves in before returning to the treatment room in hopes of seeing the light on dealing with a complication that they were left in the dark about.

DENTAL ASSISTANT (see "My Girl"): A female employee the dentist can no longer refer to as "My Girl" as in "I'll have My Girl get it" without being criticized for acting inappropriately or, even worse, having to answer to allegations of discrimination in a civil action brought against them. Sexist language and sexist behavior will not be tolerated in a dental office. You only get away with that at home.

DENTAL INSURANCE: Add a third party that you can't rely on to speak the truth about your benefits, to protect you from being discriminated against because of your preexisting condition, or to make good on the promises they ran on while lobbying for your support to elect their policy. In many ways, this party is no different in giving you the screwing over that you're already getting from the other two.

DENTAL OUTSOURCING: A cost-cutting strategy that dentists are copying from corporate America for lowering their operating expenses by subbing out whatever services they can to "those faraway places with the strange-sounding names" where the labor costs are so low that local companies can't possibly match them without going out of business.

If it takes six weeks for your dentist to get your crown back from the lab, it's a safe bet that it's probably Made in China and a sure bet that you'll never know unless you're married to the UPS delivery man.

If you have a hard time making yourself understood to the answering service operator and she asks that you please remain on hold until a supervisor can be brought on the line, your call has probably been forwarded for some international attention. This is a case where you have to go the extra mile, lots of them, to get after-hours care thanks to your stay-at-home dentist.

When relief is being outsourced, it's an internationally good idea to keep an ample supply of painkillers in your medicine cabinet.

DENTAL SPECIALIST: A dentist who can rightfully claim expert status in any of dentistry's specialties upon graduating from a postgraduate program at an accredited dental school.

The professional success of a specialist is measured not in the time it takes to demonstrate their clinical expertise—that's a given, but only half the job. Where the rubber meets the road is how effectively they use their time kissing up to the local general dentists for patient referrals under the Food for Referrals Entitlement Act. A specialist's subspecialty becomes making lunch reservations, ordering as many compliments (as opposed to condiments) as it takes to feed his prospect's ego, all in the hopes of earning the just desserts he feels entitled to. A Food for Thought Exchange, on the other hand, is of little interest to the specialist unless it's the dentist feeding off his ideas to satisfy an appetite for filling him with as many referrals as possible.

DENTAL TEAM: A broad-reaching (no pun intended) reference to the women who coexist in the office. That a cooperative and productive work environment dedicated to exceeding patients' expectations with knock-your-socks-off service occurs comes only by accident. Most dental teams are made up of individual position players who between the constant back biting among themselves look for any opportunity to pull the dentist aside to complain how "no one does anything around here except me."

Leaving dentists with the same unanswered question that mystified Rodney King: Why can't they just get along?

DISAPPOINTMENT BOOK: The book that's left after the receptionist has finished applying whiteout on the scheduled appointments that have been cancelled in the original Appointment Book. Whoever is the bearer of these bad tidings will most likely get the blame, which explains why most receptionists ask the new girl to deliver it.

DRIVE-THRU DENTAL CENTERS: Using the fast-food model to provide service with a smile, deliver it to you in the comfort of your own car, and guarantee that you'll never pay more than the fee that's posted, what's NOT to like about getting dentistry "your way"? You don't even have to bother making an appointment. All you need to do is show up when you're in the mood, make your selection from the menu of services offered, make full payment at the first window, drive up to the treatment station at the next window, put your head on the headrest, and "open your mouth and say ah" (lyrics from the song "Little Shop of Horrors").

This concept has dentists salivating at the thought of getting paid in advance and no longer being left holding the bag filled with overdue bills. That's for Whoppers if we're talking Burger King.

Necessity is the mother of invention, which is why the convenience of a drive-thru makes a lot of $ense for whoever figures out how to set it up.

E

ENCORE: A request made by an adoring patient as soon as her dentist's treatment performance is coming to an end, pleading for him to stick with the "drill." The chances of a dentist returning to the treatment room in response to the cries of "please, please, please do another tooth" from a patient who just can't get enough fall somewhere between fat and none. If you are never satisfied with the amount of time spent in the capable hands of your dentist, you are in need of some professional help—just not more of his.

EVIDENCE-BASED DENTISTRY (EBD): A newly minted term referring to the scientific body of facts (including but not limited to examination findings, x-rays, clinical notes, intraoral photographs, medical and dental health questionnaires, as well as summaries of treatment performed in other offices) that the profession came up with which makes it harder for a patient to voice their objection to recommended treatment without sounding like a dummy. Why are you hearing the term EVB now? Was there something your dentist was missing when he made the diagnosis that he based your treatment on in the past? Of course not, except that since many dentists were having trouble selling the results to fill their appointment books, maybe using terms like EVB to eliminate any doubts would. I'm not buying it as anything other than an idea that should have been DOA when it first came under consideration.

EXPERT: The status that any dentist who is more than fifty miles from his office can claim in anything just by saying so. Once past the Fifty-Mile Limit, "professional license" can be taken to exaggerate unrivaled proficiency and expertise in everything except running on time, because if he does, no one will believe anything he says ever again.

F

FOOD FOR REFERRALS: The Entitlement Act that specialists hope to benefit from by taking a potential referral source to lunch at a restaurant where the prices are so high that they feel entitled to be the beneficiary of additional referrals. The specialists I polled felt it would be unprofessional, if not rude, for the next few specialty cases after taking a dentist to lunch to be referred to anyone except them. A sincere "thank you" simply doesn't fill the bill, or pay for it, which is why the fees anticipated from treating the dentist's patients are counted on. There has been much discussion over whether the success rate of these Referral Wine & Dines are proportional to the amount spent hosting them. Most of the dentists I polled refused to comment on anything so "ludicrously unprofessional." A small minority, under the condition of anonymity, said they couldn't really answer until after they had a chance to look at the menu.

FORENSIC DENTISTRY: The art and science of identifying the deceased (the corpse) by comparing all available dental records after conducting a postmortem clinical examination of the remains. There is one exception, not worthy of even being mentioned but nonetheless added because I was a witness to it.

This is the case of an "esteemed" dental school classmate who continued treatment on a patient who had died. He didn't understand the difference between dead and very cooperative when someone keeps their mouth wide open for two hours without taking a single breath.

Presumably he does now. No longer engaging in Forensic Dentistry, my former colleague is currently limiting his practice to live patients in an affluent suburb outside New York City.

G

GIFT WRAPPING: The extensive use of dental plaques in decorating office walls to create the impression, whether accurate or misplaced, that the dentist's accomplishments are substantial. The generous use of mounting credentials for public view is intended to give patients a sense of security, confirming that they have come not just to the right place, but to the *best* place. Whether it's to create a false sense or makes real sense is open to interpretation. To those who say you can't put lipstick on a pig, I'm saying that it all depends on the shade applied.

H

HEART MURMUR: The two words on a health questionnaire that, should a patient admit to having only "a little one," can result in a lifetime Rx for antibiotics before all dental treatment, cleanings too. The preventive dose protects the patient from the bacteria in their saliva getting into the bloodstream and doing damage, causing a serious heart problem. This is a prescription for prevention for the dentist as well, protecting him from liability in the statistically unlikely event that a patient reporting any murmur actually has one or one that calls for an antibiotic to be taken.

If in doubt, it's safer for a patient to take the Fifth, because anything said that suggests the remote possibility of having a heart murmur carries a lifetime sentence for taking medicine for all future appointments until the day a cardiologist's letter says different.

In the absence of a reprieve, you will be forced to endure a protocol that guarantees to keep you in a chronic State of Overmedication, which is potentially more hazardous to your health than the majority of heart murmurs that patients walk in with but haven't admitted to.

HIRING: A process which most dentists have no training in or prior experience with that's to blame for offices "manned" by women who aren't fit to work there. The best that most clueless dentists can hope for when hiring someone is bad luck, which is a lot better than no luck at all.
As someone with two ex-wives on his resume, I know firsthand what having no luck in making choices is all about.

HOUSE CALLS: The trips real doctors (usually an MD) make to administer to patients at their homes which are usually telegraphed when all of the hand towels in the bathroom are replaced with clean ones. The only house calls the majority of dentists make are the ones at the end of the day to their significant others, warning them that they are on the way home.

I

IMPLANTS: Not the ones filled with silicone or saline, but just like them, placed under the skin to improve the quality of life of the recipient. Titanium substitute roots are surgically placed in either upper or lower jaws and, after the several months it takes to attach to the bone (osseointegrate), will be uncovered and used as anchors for permanent crowns or bridges. The ultimate second chance that, like most, costs more than doing what you could have done in the first place and saved yourself a lot of time and money, not to mention the swelling.

INSIDER TRADING: The non-prosecuted practice of trading on the privileged information obtained behind your dentist's back to uncover the name of his. Having your records transferred there once you do should pay off because, after all, if he's your dentist's top choice, shouldn't he become yours?

INTRAORAL CAMERA: A camera that has its lens embedded in a portable wand for capturing images inside the mouth that can be stored, printed as a photo, or displayed on a computer monitor. This allows you to see what the dentist does, theoretically getting you on the "same page" for seeing the problem, making the explanation of what it takes to fix it a whole lot easier.

If only what it takes to fix it is really what it takes. Perception can be "doctored" to create an image that is no reflection of reality. That doesn't mean that seeing isn't to be believed. It's just that while some pictures may be worth a thousand words, there are others that can be described by one: fake.

J

JOSE CANSECO: A baseball professional who, unlike his dental counterparts, was punished for engaging in performance-enhancement activities instead of congratulated for partaking in them.

JULES (MISTER): The Father of PM (Push Merchandise), who I credit for losing the "g" on "stunning," giving birth to the salesmanship closing exclamation for the ages, and for earning the extra commission from pushing the shoes marked with a PM out the door. What I learned from Mister Jules became the foundation upon which I built a case acceptance technique for pushing patients out the door with my recommendation for stunnin' makeovers fresh in their minds, but not before making the appointment to begin treatment.

K

KICKBACK: The "vig" that's legal for a lawyer to request from another in exchange for referring a client. A kickback can range from a nominal percentage of the total fees charged to one that even a loan shark from Boston's North End would be too embarrassed to ask for.

General dentists, on the other hand, are prohibited from asking or receiving anything other than the token thank you (holiday rhododendrons and Harry & David fruit baskets a given) for referring a patient to a specialist without suffering recriminations. This explains why a referring dentist has no qualms about ordering the most expensive item on the menu when they go out to lunch with a specialist.

L

LACKIMONY: The condition of financial inadequacy calling for those patients so afflicted to be calling their dentist to postpone their appointment for elective cosmetic dentistry until such time that they go into remission. It's no different than a disenfranchised spouse who doesn't put the alimony check in the mail. The reason in both cases is clear; it's that the check written to satisfy either obligation won't. The prognosis, even for the most advanced cases, is for a complete cure once $ucce$$ful Infu$ion therapy has been administered.

LAUGHING GAS: A mixture of nitrous oxide and oxygen gases inhaled by the patient through a nosepiece that when judiciously administered by the dentist (with a dental assistant present) is the most effective and safest way to eliminate a patient's anxiety—notwithstanding the remote possibility that this sense of security felt while being drilled on "under the influence" could turn out to be a false one. If given injudiciously, the gases can escape to give the dentist and his assistant an inadvertent "buzz" that will not only reduce their anxiety but cause them to forget to monitor the nitrous oxide/oxygen mixture you are inhaling. The consequences can be as serious as allowing the safe analgesia level to progress to anesthesia, a state where the patient won't be able to breathe on their own. There won't be anything to laugh about if you never regain consciousness.

LEAD POISONING: Something that has always been a cause for concern when you stick a lead pencil in your finger or before you move into an old house that might have lead paint. The metal poisoning debate about the potentially harmful side effects of toxic substances leaking from mercury-containing "silver" fillings, ones that can be found in just about anyone who has ever been to the dentist, shows no signs of resolution. The final verdict is still out, but not the one issued by State Boards of Dentistry, which resulted in a number of dentists losing their license to practice. Organized dentistry was making an example of any charlatan who dared to challenge the safety of mercury use in the oral cavity. Any dentists caught warning their patients of the potentially harmful side effects of mercury leaking from the metal fillings (which they were recommending be replaced with either gold or composite resin) were taken to the proverbial woodshed and left out to dry.

Such was the animosity in the profession, that if this had occurred during the Old Wild West, the bullets in their backs would be the only lead poisoning these "pioneers" would have to worry about.

LIP SERVICE: See CUSTOMER SERVICE to learn why you're getting this instead of that.

LITTLE SHOP OF HORRORS: What began as an Off Broadway musical about an abusive dentist(depicted as if there are any other kind) who got what he deserved courtesy of a self-inflicted overdose of nitrous oxide from his recreational use of 'laughing gas', that quite frankly scared the daylights out of all the dentists who do. The unprofessional use of nitrous oxide was dramatically reduced right after the movie version came out and the Steve Martin (the dentist) scene where he dies because he can't get the mask off his face hit a little too close to the office.

Home may be where the heart is, but there's no better place like home for getting high.

LITTLE PEGS: What patients call what's left of the teeth after their dentist drills them down to make a crown.

While dentists prefers to sugarcoat the massive reductions by characterizing these teepee-shaped little pegs as "preparations," the fact that what's left looks more like the last bite of a sugar cone makes this explanation a little hard to swallow.

M

MADE IN CHINA: The words you won't find engraved on the inside of any crown that your dentist outsources to a Chinese dental laboratory, which in itself would explain why it takes six
weeks to get your case back, giving a whole new meaning to "takeout."

MAGNIFICATION: What your dentist ought to be using while performing your treatment. Magnification is easily accomplished when he wears custom magnification glasses that allow him to zoom in on the operating field and see what he would have missed if he had settled for his perfect 20-20 vision.

This is the ultimate "I" protection[7] you should, even at the risk of sounding argumentative, insist on before any dental treatment is begun.

MALPRACTICE INSURANCE: Liability protection that a DMD has to pay a lot less for than an MD based on the insurance industry's experience with settling claims resulting from a dentist's error in judgment (screw-up)—which pales in comparison to what it costs when an RD (real doctor) does. Unlike the history of generous medical settlements that made personal liability lawyers rich, their clients "made whole," and a number of insurance companies paying off the judgments declare bankruptcy, selling dental liability policies makes whoever does a lot of money because actual claims are few and far between. Dentists are allergic to admitting mistakes, preferring to connect the rash of complications to the "complexity of the case," which is tantamount to saying "I don't make any." Unlike medicine, dentists perform their treatment in the protected setting of a private office, where the only ones looking over their shoulder are dental assistants, and they are the only ones writing "whatever it takes" in the record to cover themselves.

This is a policy of personal liability protection that only a dentist can sell to himself, one that comes without paying a premium, but one that comes at a cost.

McDENTAL: see Drive-Thru Dentistry

MERCURY POISONING: see Lead Poisoning

---

[7] This opinion is mine and mine alone, and in no way is meant to cast aspersions on the judgment of any dental professional, the accuracy of his technique, or the quality of his treatment for practicing without it. The only exception I'd make for allowing another dentist to work on me without it would be one wearing a cape with a large letter "S" emblazoned across his blue clinic top.

MINIMALLY INVASIVE DENTISTRY (MID): A term conceived to sell patients on dental treatment by correcting the mistaken impression that wholesale tooth reduction, such as grinding down teeth to little pegs (for crowns), is routine.

You can fool some of the patients some of the time, but not many of them are fool enough to believe this term, which is probably why its use for putting a kinder and gentler face on the dental experience has disappeared.

MINUTE: What the dentist tells you will only hurt for one that you're better off using a sundial to measure.

MONEY JOINT: A term of affection given by personal liability lawyers who make their bones suing dentists, for the TMJ and its history of paying them off big-time in malpractice cases.

This fairly new profit center for Members of the Cloth was spelled out in a daylong seminar for lawyers allegedly called "Making the Money Joint Click for You." The attendees were instructed on how to argue "irreversible jaw pain" by choosing from a *dental treatment gone wrong* list to make their case. The TMJ doesn't print money; it just makes it for them.

N

NEEDLEPHOBIC: The term characterizing those who, so horrified at the thought of getting a shot, will only seek dental care when the physical pain of a toothache becomes more than they can take. It can be such an overwhelming emotional buildup that many so afflicted routinely faint after receiving an injection, no matter that they didn't feel it. On the plus side, this serves as a deterrent to an IV-facilitated drug habit.

O

ODENTALCARE: The improbable takeoff from the Marine slogan of leaving no smile behind to get your vote. The probable takeoff being if it doesn't put a smile on your face, you are probably a Republican.

P

PAIN: What your dentist promises will only hurt for a minute (see MINUTE), which ranks as the next greatest lie after "I'm from the government and I'm here to help you." If the shoe were on the other foot, most dentists I know wouldn't open their mouths for anything other than asking for more Novocain and making their dentist wait until it takes effect before reopening.

PATOS (Payment at the Time of Service): The gift that's on every dentist's Christmas Wish List, that no matter how carefully he writes it, no matter that he's checked it twice, won't be forthcoming anytime soon. The unmitigated nerve of your dentist's receptionist in asking for it is strictly BH.

Bah Humbug.

PATIENT RECORD: A written (or printed) description of your treatment that we rely on your dentist to enter accurately. A patient record, unlike history, can't be trusted to the future for being rewritten, which is why some dentists go through great lengths to make sure anything that might reflect poorly on their judgment won't be any part of it. It's the telling words of advice from the ER nurse before I made my entry in the hospital chart that comes to mind: "Doctor, just remember, write whatever it takes to cover yourself." In legalese *res ipsa loquitur* translates to "the facts speak for themselves," ones that won't be speaking if they're not recorded.

PEER REVIEW: A voluntary option offered by most dental societies for a committee made up of local dentists (peers) to investigate a patient's complaint and mediate an equitable settlement to circumvent a lawsuit. This appointed committee, doctored by generalists and specialists, conducts its own fact-finding investigation to get to the root of the problem, beginning with an examination of the patient and a review of everything in her record. What happens next is an interview with the accused before going into Executive Session to deliberate. (Coincidentally, more than half the complaints made involve problems originating from a "failed" root canal.)

The committee's nonbinding recommendation, for which they are held harmless, is presented to both parties, either of whom may take it, leave it, litigate it, or as one disenchanted dentist told his peers, "shove it." Does this work? Can the decision be impartial? Put it this way; if the case happens to involve a dentist who doesn't refer his patients to local specialists, his chances of getting the benefit of a doubt are a definite maybe.

I'm not suggesting that a lack of familiarity breeds contempt. I'm promising that by the time this process runs its course, of that there will be no doubt. This illustrates how the ties that bind in nonbinding arbitration are strictly arbitrary, as is the decision for who gets to be set loose.

PLAQUE: What most dental patients call the film of bacteria that clings to the walls of their teeth that hygienists don't remove until "shoulding" on them for not doing as good a job as they should for keeping their mouth clean. To avoid a hygienist's Plaque Attack, more patients fail to respond to the "long overdue for a cleaning and checkup" reminder to skip the lecture on what a dirty mouth they have. They can get that from their significant other without even having to make an appointment. One variation that falls under the dentist's *best-kept secret* category refers to plaque(s) as professionally framed certificates of recognition that while sharing the similar clinging affinity of the bacteria in the saliva are found on office walls, not the enamel ones.

This variety of plaques on the walls may give you a false sense of well-being, while any appearing on the enamel needs to be taken off before any such assurance of well-being can be given. The total effect of wall-to-wall plaques can be hard to take, but shouldn't ever be taken at face value without doing a little discovery.

PREAPPROVAL: Something every married man has to get from his wife before making a decision, which doesn't excuse him from getting the blame if it turns out to be the wrong one. The dentist's insignificant other's insurance company demands nothing less. These not-for-any-one-else's-profit-except-their-own won't pay a claim for treatment, no matter that it's covered under the policy, without receiving a "prior approved" from a claims examiner sitting at a desk thousands of miles away. No matter that they know nothing about dentistry; all they need to know is what to look for to delay approvals from being issued.

PRE-DOCTOR (PD): The designation assigned to anyone with a plan, no matter how remote, of applying to a school of higher learning, whether on a campus, on the internet, or on a television correspondence network authorized to confer a degree which includes the word "doctor."

PREMEDICATION: A controlled substance prescribed by the dentist to a patient, occasionally dispensed to himself and his dental assistant to insure that the treatment experience will be relaxing and stress-free for everyone. This could be where the expression "feeling no pain" was conceived.

PROFESSIONAL COURTESY: A fee discount for professional services given by one doctor to another, not so much because they are special friends, but to perpetuate the myth that turnabout being fair play will play into sparing each other's pocketbook when the operating tables, so to speak, are turned. These magnanimous gestures are more like disingenuous ones, given that the doctor's "professional courtesy" is passed on as fee increases to all the other patients to make up the difference. While the professionals continue to get it, it's the doctor giving it who gets all the credit. The only thing you get is to pay for it.

How courteous can that be?

PRO-CHOICE: The choice made by a patient to extract a tooth that could have been saved which, in the absence of a pro-root-canal crowd forming a human chain around an oral surgery dental clinic to prevent her entry, is accomplished without getting into a fight.

PROPHYLAXIS: Dentistry's word for playing it safe, accomplished by coming in to have your teeth cleaned and checked—a word that sounds similar to the rubber protection one buys for better being safe than sorry.

PUSH MERCHANDISE (PM): The designation assigned to goods or services that a salesman gets an added bonus for pushing out the door on, in, or with a satisfied customer. What began as code for the extra commission earned for pushing out as many of last year's high fashion shoes as possible became the on-the-job training I received at Mister Jack's Shoe Boutique that enabled me to "push out" my profession's PM, cosmetic dentistry. I decided it would be better not to push my luck and come out with a personal epiphany, one of the reasons I published this book under a pseudonym.

Q

Q SCHOOL: A takeoff on how golfing professionals get 'qualified' to perform on the Main Tour that would require dentists to demonstrate their ability to consistently sell enough cosmetic dentistry before they are deemed eligible to move up to the "show." I contend that anyone with the talent to overcome the resistance of a customer to sell them a pair of shoes they never asked for, didn't want, and didn't initially see the value in will pass with flying colors. Such a dentist will have no problem earning more than enough to thrive, graduating as a "made" man and a man armed with the necessary communication skills for making a patient an offer they can't refuse.

R

REAL DOCTOR (RD): All doctors are not created equal, as the rest of us carrying anything other than the alphabet-winning letters M and D running consecutively and uninterrupted after our names are reminded. This distinction is one that most mothers would like clarity on before being introduced to their son or daughter's fiancé in order to avoid the embarrassment of having to ask: So, are you a real doctor… or just a dentist?

RECALL NOTICE: The postcard depicting someone looking under the hood of a shiny convertible with the caption "Please Call to Schedule a Return Visit"—either a reminder for a cleaning and a checkup from your dentist or the official notification from your car dealership to make an appointment to have a defective part replaced. It's no wonder dentists are referred to as "molar mechanics."

REFERRAL: The "second thought that is invariably wiser" that, with one notable exception, the doctor carries through on when he sends his patient to a specialist for the treatment he would have liked to perform (and charge for) if his ability matched his ambition. The potential for recapturing lost income when his appointment book has been decimated by whiteout opens the door to making that notable exception, breaking the promise all of us made to ourselves when we graduated dental school to never attempt treatment we weren't completely confident in our ability to complete. Necessity once again proves itself to be the Mother of Invention, which is what the dentist who finds himself in over his head will find necessary to invent an excuse as to why he didn't refer the patient to a specialist in the first place. That's when he finds himself with no choice but to come up with a mother of an explanation to save face.

REFERRAL FEE: see KICKBACK

RESTROOM: A centrally located patient bathroom that, if able to be locked from the outside after you close the door, becomes a true "place of rest," a valuable tool for the dentist who fails to resolve a life-threatening emergency. What's so critical, aside from the declining condition of the patient, are the instructions he gives to the receptionist for not calling 911 until the patient has been safely secured in the restroom.

I take no credit for this tasteless bathroom humor; that's reserved for the oral surgeon who taught my course in Emergency Medicine at dental school. He referred to this as comic relief, using the restroom as a place where the dentist could *relieve* himself from having to explain how a patient died in his office. While I doubt you find anything about his dark humor amusing, it might not be a bad idea to make a pit stop and check that your dentist's bathroom door can't be locked from the outside.

ROOT CANAL: The sterile intercourse that takes place within the thin, dark, narrow canals of the tooth roots by the action of rigid files moving back and forth, in and out. Once the hard files have finished preparing the root canal, essentially endodontic foreplay, it's now ready to be filled with a pre-fit rod of an inert filler (gutta percha), heated until it becomes soft, mixed with a sealer, and pushed under pressure to the tip of the canal.

Patients have characterized having a root canal as such an unbearable form of torture that they would willingly endure just about anything else you could think of in its place. Getting tired of hearing how "I'd rather have a baby than a root canal" by untold numbers of childbearing women in my practice, I took it upon myself to find out once and for all if they were lying. I obtained a local hospital's approval to conduct my research project at their "birthing place," one that came to a quick end when I fainted within minutes of hearing the first horrific screams of an expectant mother suffering excruciating labor pain.

The conclusion: Any woman who thinks that going through labor without being totally anesthetized is less painful than having root canal therapy is in for a huge surprise. In the words of the president of Men's Wearhouse (recently fired): I absolutely guarantee it!

RUBBER DAM: Dentistry's latex prophylactic, put on by your dentist before entering the oral cavity to prevent the leakage of body fluids (your saliva) from contaminating the operating field. And while it's not a lay-up to physically put one on, it's harder than a slam dunk unless you're at least 6'5" to keep it on over the course of an appointment. Nonetheless, it's worthwhile doing whatever it takes because it's better (to be) safe than sorry. So it's damned when you do, damned if you don't.

S

SEMI-NONFICTION: The genre I chose for writing this book that gave me artistic license to stretch the truth and make it easier for you to swallow. Using semi-truths to expose heretofore "truths used and abused" for selling you on elective cosmetic dentistry is simply priceless. Using your MasterCard to pay for a copy of *Confessions of a Cosmetic Dentist* represents a fraction of the price it costs for a full smile makeover, which, once you've read it cover to cover, will protect you from swallowing a case presentation hook, line, and sinker.

SLEEP DENTISTRY: The sweet dream "to die for" to escape the pain and suffering of dental treatment that's given fearful dental patients something to live for. The marketing campaigns promising to make your dreams come true are aimed at the lifetime dental phobic who would just as soon pay double for a body double to take their place to get the work done. That this option has not always been a lifesaver for those needing it is something YOU should be losing sleep over before agreeing to have it.

Standing in the way of delivering predictable and safe experiences are the increasing numbers of dentists offering sleep dentistry with nothing more than a weekend course on their résumé and nothing more than a certificate for doing less than nothing to earn it. The three-day course in Conscious Sedation I attended at a prominent dental school continuing education center, given by an esteemed member of the faculty and author of a book on the same subject, taught me all I needed to know: NEVER put anyone to sleep when you've only been given fifteen minutes of troubleshooting on what to do if they aren't waking up.

Sleep dentistry is the nightmare you might never wake up from if your dentist got his degree at one of these three-day colleges of anesthesiology.

STANDARD OF CARE: Something you shouldn't have to worry about when you get dental treatment—except you do. The difference between good and good enough won't make as much of a difference as the one between standard and substandard, all of which you rely on your dentist to take into account before bringing your seat to the upright position.

STUNNIN': The Gold Standard for selling anything to anybody summed up in a word: stunnin'—what's left after you lose the "g" from "stunning." Credit for bastardizing this highly complimentary adjective for proclaiming magnificence belongs to Mister Jules, a slight-of-build, balding senior shoe salesman extraordinaire at Mister Jack's, an upscale women's shoe boutique in Short Hills, NJ. It was there, laboring part time under the pseudonym of Mister Alan while attending Seton Hall's Graduate School of Biology, that I made my bones in salesmanship, so to speak, not to mention some extra money.

It's accurate to say that what I learned from Mister Jules, who I nominate as The Father of Push Merchandise, outweighs the sum total of all the knowledge imparted to me in my twenty-four months of breast cancer research. A striking figure, Mister Jules had the minimum amount of gray scraggly hair, which he was able to tie back in a wispy ponytail with his nicotine-stained but professionally manicured, arthritic fingers.

His legendary response to "Well, Jules, tell me the truth, do you really like the way they look on my feet?" from a client trying on a PM (the two letters that earn you an added bonus on top of the standard ten percent commission for pushing any merchandise so designated out the door) was as predictable as an alimony check being cashed. What else BUT "stunnin'," as in what's not to like about ringing the register on an added commission of $25 to $50.

I put the word on the shelf until I graduated from dental school, and began using it as soon as I opened my practice: My promise for how stunnin' their new smile would look pushed so many smiles out the door of my small office within that first year, I had to hire an associate and build a new office twice the size of my first. You wouldn't expect anything less from anyone lucky enough to get the word from The Father of Push Merchandise.

T

TALK: As in "Can I talk to you for a minute?" When spoken by a dental assistant closing the door to the dentist's private office at the end of the day, it usually means she is about to give her notice. And that means there's nothing more to talk about.

TMJ (short for temporomandibular joint): see MONEY JOINT

TREATMENT CON$ULTATION: An appointment that gives your dentist the opportunity to sit knee to knee and eye to eye across the table from you to present a list of treatment recommendations that you don't want to hear, don't believe you need, don't want to be talked into, and don't want to pay for even if you can. Dentists on a mission to sell you Appearance Dentistry come prepared with a script. A game plan they probably got from a Practice Management seminar where motivational speakers (like me) send course participants home with a cookbook of recipes and specific baking instructions for taking your "temperature" to ask for treatment acceptance only when they're sure it's "well done."

Why do dentists take courses on how to sell cosmetic dentistry? It's largely because dental schools never expected that their graduates would need to learn how to sell anything.

U

UNWRITTEN CODE: The omertà of the non-wise guy's profession that's not a code of silence honored between doctors for keeping quiet to avoid bad-mouthing the work of another brother. There may be honor among thieves, but there's no love lost practicing in a profession where never having to say "I'm sorry" as you climb over the backs of the competition is pretty much the norm.

UNDIVIDED ATTENTION: What you don't get when your dentist divides his time among the other patients he's scheduled along with you. One way for getting him to pay some would be asking his receptionist for the group therapy rate the next time the appointment that's been reserved for you is part of a group reservation.

V

VENEEREMIA (aka The Big V): A condition synonymous with porcelain insufficiency resulting from an inadequate number of porcelain laminate veneers in the oral cavity, which for a select group of cosmetic dentists is only adequate once they've been placed on every tooth. Veneeremia is a condition that's completely reversible with early treatment, which could begin as early as tomorrow if your dentist can fit you into his schedule.

W

WAITING LIST: This is a list that patients ask to be put on indicating their willingness to drop everything they are doing at a moment's notice should an earlier appointment become available. What's common for scheduling your first appointment with a primary care physician could be nothing further from the truth in The People's Republic of Dental America. The only waiting that dental patients wanting to schedule cosmetic dentistry will encounter is the time it takes to decide which one of them the receptionist has available for tomorrow to take. Those waiting on a list for a kidney, liver, or a heart should only be so lucky.

WHITEOUT: What was used prior to the computer delete key for altering a patient's record to avoid blame for a "complication." And blamed is what a dentist should be if he doesn't apply some to escape what he would be held accountable for if it can be seen in black and white.

Hindsight may be 20-20, but doctoring history comes with the foresight of sparing yourself from ever having to rewrite it.

X

X-RAYS: The pictures of your teeth taken with an X-ray machine that your dentist needs the light of an illuminated view box to read. Despite being told that the amount of radiation you're exposed to is less than what you get by standing in the sun, you have to wonder how safe it really is when the assistant covers you from head to toe with lead aprons before running out of the room and hiding behind a lead-lined wall before unleashing some of that harmless "sun" on the film.

Y

YELLOW PAGES: An added section of annually published book of business listings that the telephone company's sales representatives try to sell dentists increasingly larger advertising space in, now that the primitive advertising restrictions for professionals have been lifted. From prohibited, to discouraged, to regulated, to frowned upon, local dental societies haven't been bashful about calling serial advertisers on the carpet to answer for anything they deemed unprofessional.

As a dentist who was the first in my less-than-cosmopolitan and sparsely populated peninsula to make a splash with a full-page display ad in the local Yellow Pages, I liken the waves created from the aftershocks once the book made land as nothing less than tsunami-like.

Z

If you've followed the alphabet trail through the Definitions You Won't Find Anywhere Else (that when you read you'll know why) you've now come to Z End of the book, which brings you to A new beginning. You now have the good sense to recognize when to get off the tracks in time to avoid getting run over by your dentist's cosmetic enthusiasm. You can no longer be blinded by the bonding light, now that you've been…enlightened.

"There is no knowledge that is not power."
—Ralph Waldo Emerson, American essayist and poet